At Home in Your Body

How the Gospel Quiets the Noise & Transforms Our Views of Health, Beauty, & Body Image

Ashley Nicole Hoover

At Home in Your Body
Copyright © 2025 by Ashley Nicole Hoover

Library of Congress Cataloging-in-Publication Data

LCCN: 2025926706 (paperback) ISBN: 978-1-961732-31-5 (ebook) | ISBN: 978-1-961732-30-8 (paperback) | ISBN: 978-1-961732-29-2 (hardcover)

Scripture quotations unless otherwise marked have been taken from the Christian Standard Bible®, Copyright © 2017 by Holman Bible Publishers. Used by permission. Christian Standard Bible® and CSB® are federally registered trademarks of Holman Bible Publishers.

Any internet addresses (website, blogs, etc.) and telephone numbers in this book are offered as a resource. They are not intended in any way to be or imply an endorsement from Called Creatives Publishing, nor does Called Creatives Publishing vouch for the content of these sites and numbers for the life of this book.

Published in association with Called Creatives Publishing, www.calledcreativespublishing.com

Cover Design: Called Creatives Publishing
Interior Design: Called Creatives Publishing
Interior Formatting: Dallas Hodge

Dedication

For my Thursday night crew:
Allison, Lara, Lindsy, Rez & Sarah—
Thank you for believing in this before I did.
For the prayers, the edits, the laughter,
and the steady call to keep going.
You've encouraged me to live out the gospel in real life,
every single week spent at our table.

Contents

Part 3 - The Eternal Body

Introduction

Every August, I prepare our home for a new year of homeschool. I purchase curriculum, clear out clutter from our space, and think about all the goals I have for the next season. Part of that ritual includes rereading a small book called *Teaching from Rest*. Every year, without fail.

Why? Because in the shuffle of math books, literature lists, and goals for the year, I sometimes lose sight of the bigger vision. I need a reminder to return and remember.

That little book realigns my heart. It reminds me I didn't choose to homeschool because I needed my boys to master certain math facts or impress anyone with their grasp of history. The choice was never about the outcomes. It was always about faithfulness—about shaping hearts to love Christ and love learning. It's about who they are becoming, not what they can accomplish.

Before I launch into a new year, I need that reminder. I need to come home to the reason why.

And I've realized: we need a similar return when it comes to our bodies.

We know the truth—we are image bearers, made good by a good Creator. There's no doubt that there's value in caring for our bodies. But somewhere along the way, under the noise of programs, products, pressures, and promises, we lose the vision. We lose the *why*. We gather all the tools. We chase all the advice. But sometimes, we miss the forest for the trees.

My prayer is that this book will be a return and a reminder for you. The exhale you've needed. A clear window into why we care for our bodies and how we do it in a way that feels like clarity in a world that feels contradictory and confusing.

Along the way, we'll also learn to recognize the messages that distort how we see and care for our bodies—to think critically about them, to speak truth over them, and to remember the story we actually belong to.

I hope you come back to it whenever you need it. Because we forget. Because we are people who need to be reminded by one another, over and over, of the truest things.

I didn't write this to tell you that you're doing it all wrong. There are plenty of books that will hand you a list of fixes. I wrote this as a heart-to-heart. To remind you of Who you belong to—and how the Gospel changes *everything*.

Part 1
The Biblical Body

Our ideas about our own bodies
interact with ideas we have about Jesus's body.

— Kelly M. Kapic, *You're Only Human*

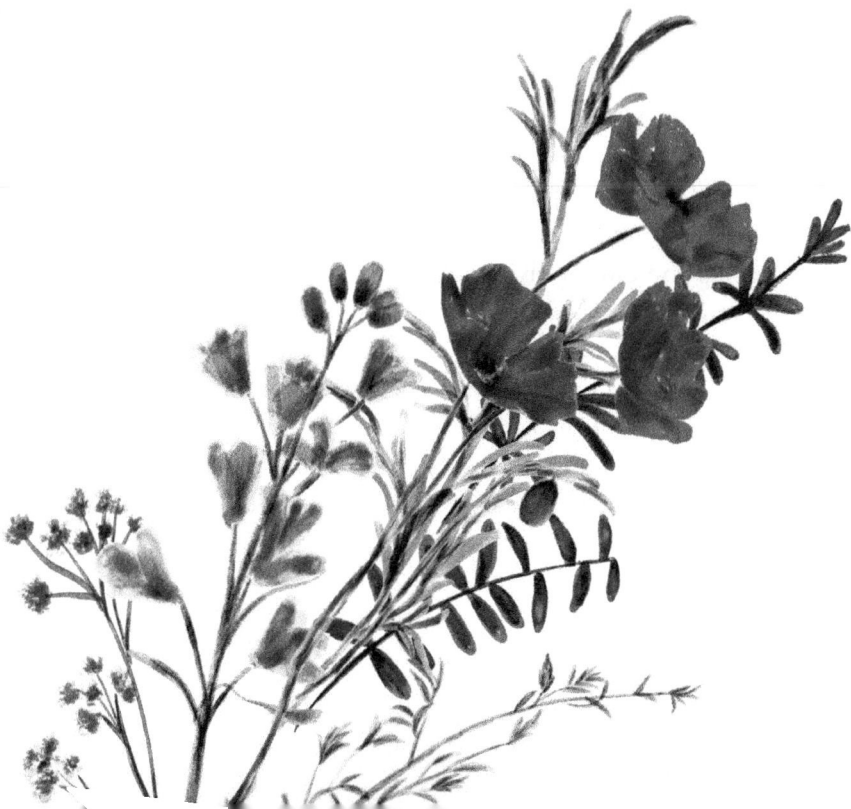

1

Body Image

Why don't we like our bodies?

Hard though it may be for us to understand,
God meant for us to have our particular body. Your body is a gift.

—Sam Allberry, *What God Has to Say About Our Bodies*

I t started with an offhand comment.

I became aware of my body in second grade. In a flurry of excitement, I slipped into a new dance costume for the yearly recital. It was a vibrant reddish-orange leotard with yellow and orange fringe, crisscrossing just above and below my torso, framing my 8-year-old belly. As I twirled around, eager for approval, a solitary comment lingered in the air: *"The costumes aren't very flattering."*

Though the words were aimed at the costume design, all I could hear was a subtle critique of my body: *it should be different, or it should be hidden.* My belly was on display in a way that, note taken, was unappealing.

I had been in tap and ballet combo classes since I was 5 years old, watching the older girls get to learn dances more like the ones I saw in Paula Abdul videos. The 80's were something. It was big hair, bright colors, and the BEST dance moves if you ask me. The Moonwalk, Roger Rabbit, the Snake, anything from the Thriller music video … need I say more?

At age 8, I was finally old enough to sign up for jazz classes. I had been looking forward to this since the day I stepped into the dance studio. But the thing I remember most about that first year was that neon, fringed costume … *that wasn't very flattering.*

That comment flipped a switch in my mind that never turned off. It became the quiet start to years of shame, frustration, and the perpetual feeling of discomfort in my skin that was only reinforced by a string of similar stories. It was like always wearing clothing that never fit quite right. I always wished things were flatter, thinner, more toned, and more aesthetically "beautiful." What little girl doesn't want to be beautiful?

It felt normal to constantly look at my reflection and photographs and pick apart what wasn't flattering. There was me, and then there was the reflection of me, and we were enemies.

I began coping with frustrations about my body by striving to fix what I perceived as flaws, endlessly chasing some arbitrary ideal in my mind. Somewhere along the way, beauty got tangled up with health in a way that I have spent my entire life trying to untangle. Health was just the "healthy" way to pursue beauty. This confusion laid the foundation of my body image.

I got a job at 19 years old at a health club where I accumulated every personal training, fitness, and nutrition certification I could get. Determination drove the pursuit to educate my way to the body that I wanted (early spoiler: this did not work). A degree in health studies followed, along with coaching. Fascination with the nuances of movement led to Pilates certifications. Interest in pregnancy led to prenatal and postpartum certifications. Work continued in gyms, studios, and even included a short stint at a weight loss center. Education and experience piled up for over a decade. Every job collected another chest full of stories—women desperate for that elusive transformation that they believed would finally make them feel free and at home in their bodies. There was always something new to learn, but it never seemed to fix the problem. It was an endless dance of both love for the human body and also a hate for my own body with every bit of knowledge I gathered.

After having kids, I shifted a bit. Stress management became the thing I desperately wanted so that I could enjoy the season of life

I had always longed for. I began to care more about longevity than fitness because it was no longer just about me.

Although this transition was a step forward in some ways, it also marked my super toxic, non-toxic phase. I was scared everything would make us sick. The new mom in me was so susceptible to every marketing message that claimed everything causes cancer and that it would be my kids who would suffer. I bought every product with a label that claimed to be safe, non-toxic, organic, green, etc. My obsession with aesthetics shifted to an obsession with longevity. It was no longer just about beauty; it was about self-preservation and perfection. Still, I was trying to fix all the broken things.

The more I zoomed in and critiqued all my flaws, the more I found things I didn't like. The harder I worked, the worse my body image became. Sure, there might be temporary pride in some minor accomplishments. Still, there was never the thing I really longed for—contentment and comfort in my own skin.

We outgrow so many insecurities that we have as kids and teens, and yet, the research shows midlife women are still mostly unhappy with their bodies. In a study done with women in their 50s, only 12.2% reported satisfaction with their size. The kicker is that the article says that (1) these women tended to put considerable effort into "achieving and maintaining" their satisfaction, and (2) it didn't exclude them from being dissatisfied with other parts of their bodies.[1]

I lived in the "achieving and maintaining" cycle most of my life. It is exhausting and frustrating.

It wasn't until I approached my late 30s that I realized I had been trying to fit my view of the body, which had been shaped by a multi-billion-dollar industry, into my Christian worldview. Some of it seemed to fit and make sense. If God made our bodies, then everything we do in the name of health should be good, right?

But why did I still have so many negative feelings about my body? Why were joy, peace, and hope missing from the picture? Shouldn't

---

1 Cristin D. Runfola et al., "Characteristics of Women with Body Size Satisfaction at Midlife: Results of the Gender and Body Image (GABI) Study," *Journal of Women & Aging* 25, no. 4 (2013): 287–304, https://doi.org/10.1080/08952841.2013.816215.

the fruit of the Spirit be visible in all areas of our lives, especially in those we claim are essentially good?

These questions led me to where I am now. For the past five years, I've been asking one disruptive question: What does a truly biblical view of my body even mean?

I knew the verses. We are created in God's image (Genesis 1:27). He has declared this part of His creation *very good* (Genesis 1:31). We are fearfully and wonderfully made (Psalm 139:14). Our very body is the temple of the Holy Spirit (1 Corinthians 6:19).

But if we believe these things are true, why don't they shape how we see ourselves?

I've never met a single woman who hasn't thought something negative about her body.

Years ago, I attended a large convention, which was almost entirely made up of women. We're talking about 20,000-plus attendees. I love being at events with other women.

We got to choose our breakout sessions, and I chose one based solely on the speaker. It was overflowing, so I sat on the floor along the wall. I got out my notebook, my favorite pen, and I was ready to learn everything I could about being a great leader, marketer, and businesswoman, but she did something unexpected…

She asked us to stand up.

The room was quiet as we waited. *Where is she going with this?* She asked us to sit down if we had never thought negatively about our bodies.

Silence and stillness.

No one moved, but I felt something for sure. It was the kind of heartbreak that sits heavy in your chest and makes you just a little angry.

Her talk would hinge on relatability and how shared experiences connect us. The speaker made her point. But I don't know that I will ever be the kind of person who shrugs my shoulders and says, "Welp, that's just how it is." I am all for uniting with other women in shared experiences. But I reject that the one thing that we continually connect on is the dislike of our bodies. This? This is the commonality that spans all age groups of women from all over the country and with different backgrounds? Mention something you don't like about your body in a room full of women, and you will see how quickly everyone contributes their own grievances about their bodies. In a culture like ours, I understand how we got here. What I can't make peace with is how those of us who believe we are created in the image of a good God still echo the same sentiment.

Deep down, we know we should feel different in our bodies than we do. I look back, and I don't understand why my younger self struggled with body image because I would love to have that body now. It seems clear that it had nothing to do with my actual body but everything to do with my *beliefs* about my body. How I felt about my body was almost exclusively based on what I thought my body should look like.

This is not just an issue for women who don't like the way they look. Even if you love how you look, the challenge is that it will inevitably change. We age. We get pregnant. We get sick.

We cannot change our body image by changing what we see in the mirror.

It is an issue of placing our value in the wrong place, misunderstanding the purpose of the body, and creating habits around outward appearance to the detriment of our whole selves. When we separate our bodies from who we are, it becomes easier to stop seeing our bodies as something good.

Many of us work tirelessly to fix the problem by changing our bodies, while others focus on changing how we think about our appearance. We see this idea within the body positivity movement, which encourages celebrating all bodies, regardless of size, shape, or appearance. Perhaps in recognizing that changing our bodies doesn't solve the deeper issue, we've turned to fixing our thoughts, hoping that by declaring everything good and beautiful—terms that have become subjective in our culture—we can repair our body image.

While the heart behind the body positivity movement aims to foster love and acceptance, it falls short. There is a difference between thinking happy thoughts, reciting what we wish were true, and meditating on what is objectively, unarguably true. Simply masking our insecurities with hollow affirmations doesn't work. We are still addressing the problem at the surface without digging deep to uproot the real source of our struggle. In fact, research shows that affirmations we don't believe can actually be harmful.[2] The takeaway is simple: you cannot lie to yourself.

As Christians, our beliefs form a deeply rooted, unchanging foundation for our lives. Changing how we think about our bodies is essential, but those thoughts must overflow from our beliefs, as we are instructed to take every thought captive to Christ (2 Corinthians 10:5). **It's not enough to declare all things good and beautiful if those definitions are shaped by culture rather than our Bibles.**

So yes, we must transform the way we think, but it's not through mere positive affirmations or wishful thinking. We must ask: **What is true?** Truth is the foundation of our

> Jesus told him, "I am the way, the truth, and the life."
> —John 14:6

faith, and since Jesus is the Truth (John 14:6), He becomes the foundation for how we see our bodies. We need to go deeper than surface-level changes in behavior—we need to pull apart the puzzle pieces of our body image and reexamine our beliefs. Chances are, there are some fragments of a worldview that don't belong.

Therefore, we have to get curious and explore how the fact that Christ walked this earth in a human body (and still remains in a body) is wildly significant, and that you were formed in the very body you have for a purpose.

It means we must unwrap the profound truth that our bodies are not a problem to be solved, but a gift that allows us to image

---

2 Joanne V. Wood, W. Q. Elaine Perunovic, and John W. Lee, "Positive Self-Statements: Power for Some, Peril for Others," *Psychological Science* 20, no. 7 (July 2009): 860–866, https://doi.org/10.1111/j.1467-9280.2009.02370.x.

Christ to the world. And when we understand this gift, we will find ourselves in a place of genuine worship.

When we fix our eyes on Jesus, beauty and health are redefined into something that brings joy, peace, and a restoration of wholeness because a healthy body is good and glorifies God.

Health becomes sanctification embodied and a pursuit of what is good over what is easy.

Our bodies matter, and how we steward them matters. So, yes, we need to discuss the place of workouts, food, rest, and healthy choices in our lives, but we will do it after we unpack the truth that **the body is already good** and put health back in its proper place.

Then, you will be at home in your body, living well in it for the One who deserves all the glory.

Amen?

2
A Fractured View of the Body
What has defined our body image?

But secular worldviews do not come neatly labeled so we can easily recognize them. Instead they mutate into forms that we hardly recognize, becoming part of the very air we breathe. The most powerful worldviews are the ones we absorb without knowing it. They are the ideas nobody talks about—the assumptions we pick up almost by osmosis.

—Nancy R. Pearcey, *Love Thy Body*

The doctor's office is the one place you do not want to get bad news.

My early 20s were spent between shifts in the gym and classes in health studies—trying to fix whatever it was that I didn't like about myself. Workouts filled nearly every spare hour. Every food came with a side of fear. What once looked like discipline revealed itself later as disordered. Each new piece of knowledge became another weapon turned against my body. It was all about control.

Most of my early 20s are a blur, but this moment, when I was sitting in that doctor's office, the look on her face and the words that seemed to hang in the air are forever cemented in my mind.

"If you get married, I would recommend you start trying to have children right away. It might be difficult for you."

I thought I had outsmarted my body. I was more fit and more "disciplined." However, I had pushed my body into a state of survival, sacrificing long-term health for short-term control. *I did this to myself.*

The damage I had done to myself was real—not theoretical. *It wasn't healthy. I wasn't healthy.*

Here's something I've witnessed from the inside of the health and fitness industry: many women you watch and assume have it all together are quietly struggling with body image, too. I know them. I've learned from many of them. And like me, they often hide behind a wall of expertise.

In one study on body appearance pressure and idealization among fitness instructors, 59% of the female fitness instructors reported behaviors consistent with disordered eating.[3] Like everything, you cannot broad-brush an entire industry, but we need to be honest about what's being sold to us as healthy.

Most Christian women aren't struggling because they lack biblical knowledge. They're struggling because they've been subtly discipled by an industry that profits from their insecurity. Without even realizing it, we've adopted secular definitions of beauty and health, then dressed them in Christian language. The result? Our beliefs sound biblical, but our habits, motivations, and identity remain shaped by the culture.

This isn't just a personal struggle—it's a worldview issue. If we don't expose the false messages forming us, we'll keep trying to apply Gospel truth like a surface fix instead of letting it reshape the foundation.

Beliefs That Form Us

Most of us have a view of our bodies shaped through the health and fitness industry, which reflects our culture's worldview. We need to take a closer look at these ideas to recognize them for what they are. Bad ideas have a way of sneaking into our thoughts, and then we rehearse them in our daily habits before we even realize our loves,

---

3 Solfrid Bratland-Sanda, Merethe Pauline Nilsson, and Jorunn Sundgot-Borgen, "Disordered Eating Behavior Among Group Fitness Instructors: A Health-Threatening Secret?" *Journal of Eating Disorders* 3, no. 22 (2015), https://doi.org/10.1186/s40337-015-0059-x.

desires, and motivations are formed by something that doesn't align with our beliefs.

Natasha Crain presents the concept of worldview as like a puzzle. Our core beliefs about ourselves and the world around us are the pieces that form a unified picture. As Christians, we hold to a biblical worldview, meaning that the Word of God shapes how we see everything. Each piece of our puzzle—our beliefs, values, and actions—should fit into this larger biblical picture, forming one cohesive whole.[4]

When we talk about the body, we have to begin with what it means to be human. From a biblical perspective, this means a few foundational things:

(1) We were created by God—formed from the dust, given the breath of life, and made both body and soul, material and immaterial (Genesis 2:7).

(2) We were made in His image (Genesis 1:27).

(3) We were called very good (Genesis 1:31).

(4) Jesus affirmed the goodness of the body in the Incarnation by taking on flesh, living fully embodied, and rising again in a glorified body (Luke 24:39).

(5) And from the very beginning, we were made for relationship. "It is not good for the man to be alone" (Genesis 2:18).

In contrast, the secular worldview offers a different set of pieces, forming a puzzle of its own. It dominates the health and fitness industry, influencing our thoughts about the body and how we care for it. Broadly defined, it means "an umbrella term for a variety of worldviews that ultimately function in the same way—without a commitment to the authority of a religion and its god(s)."[5]

---

4 Natasha Crain, "Practical Tips for Teaching Kids Apologetics at Home," *The Natasha Crain Podcast*, August 24, 2021, audio, 1:16:00, https://podcasts.apple.com/us/podcast/practical-tips-for-teaching-kids-apologetics-at-home/id1550242146?i=1000532918332.

5 Natasha Crain, *Faithfully Different: Regaining Biblical Clarity in a Secular Culture* (Eugene, OR: Harvest House Publishers, 2022), 41.

It's common for us to pick up pieces of other worldviews that are inconsistent with our own. This concept of picking and choosing, whether intentional or not, is called syncretism. George Barnas research shows that 88% of U.S. adults hold to an inconsistent worldview—a mix of beliefs that may appear compatible but are rooted in entirely different truths.[6] Even when we have a biblical worldview on the core beliefs, topics like health are commonly shaped by influences inconsistent with our worldview.

Sometimes these pieces might seem like they fit, but upon deeper examination, they have created a fracture in how we view our bodies. Our bodies are good, therefore we should workout, eat right, and take care of them, right? Absolutely. But we need to ensure that the overall picture of how we view the body, the purpose of the body, and how to care for the body is formed by biblical truth and not just a brand of secular health and fitness covered in a Christian veneer.

Over and over again, we see God setting His people apart, calling them to live in ways that stand out from the world around them. It's a consistent theme throughout Scripture. **God's people are meant to reflect His holiness, often by living in ways that challenge the cultural norms of their time.**

God set Abraham apart by calling him to leave what was familiar and follow Him. His faith set a foundation for a people who would be distinct, rooted in a covenant relationship with God.

He also set the Israelites apart when he gave them the Law—not as a list of rules, but as a way of life that stood in sharp contrast to the nations around them. Their dietary restrictions, Sabbath-keeping, and the way they treated others were meant to mark them as holy, a people belonging to God.

We see this again in the life of Daniel. Living in Babylon, a culture centered on wealth, power, and idol worship, Daniel's refusal to eat the king's food or bow to Babylonian gods made his faithfulness

---

6 Barna Group, "Most Adults Feel Accepted by God, but Lack a Biblical World-view," *Barna*, March 6, 2005, https://www.barna.com/research/most-adults-feel-accepted-by-god-but-lack-a-biblical-worldview/.

visible. Even in exile, God's people were called to be holy—to live in a way that did not look like the world.

If we're tempted to think that being set apart as God's people is just Old Testament history, Jesus gives us a fresh vision of the kingdom in Matthew. It's a kingdom where the meek, the poor, the hungry, the merciful, the thirsty, and the persecuted are ... blessed. These ideas are a part of the upside-down kingdom we proclaim as followers of Jesus.

God's people were always meant to look different and to live according to His ways rather than the ways of the world. That calling is no less true today. We are set apart—not just to blend in, but to reflect God's love, holiness, and truth in a world that often goes the other direction. And this is where we reach the heart of this book: **We reflect these truths through our bodies.**

Let's examine three specific worldview differences that have resulted in us adopting a view of our bodies that has left us confused about them and, therefore, about ourselves.

Dependence on Christ

The American secular worldview champions independence. I could rewrite my story from the first chapter as a girl who took matters into her own hands, educated herself, changed her habits, and got the desired results. That's the American story, right? You are the master of your destiny. If you work hard at something, you will get what you want and be satisfied. This only works, though, if I omit the parts of the story where I was never content. All the discipline in the world couldn't quiet the ache inside me. I looked like I had it together, but I didn't feel whole. There was a low-level dissonance I couldn't shake. I never felt fully at ease in my own body.

Independence means we are free to do what we want, define things the way we want, and to be the ultimate authority over our lives. Although this can make us feel temporarily empowered because it gives us a sense of ownership over our lives, it fails us. If there is anything that has caused women to be more overwhelmed and mentally overloaded, it is the feeling that it all depends on you and you alone. In the case of our bodies, we have reduced the size of our jeans to a measure of our own competence. If the number is bigger than we think it should be, it's a failure on our part. We stockpile shame for our lack of self-control because every flaw signifies a personal failure. It becomes a constant losing battle with ourselves.

Instead, Jesus tells us to be poor in spirit, meek, and hungry. This means acknowledging we lack and **are dependent** on Christ to fill the void. This was radical when Jesus first said it, and it's still radical today. The Christian life is about dependence.

> **Instead, he emptied himself by assuming the form of a servant, taking on the likeness of humanity.**
>
> **— Philippians 2:7**

Christ, of course, is the perfect picture of this. There is a theological term called kenosis, which refers to a moment where Christ willingly emptied Himself. (See Philippians 2:7: "Instead, he emptied himself, by assuming the form of a servant, being born in the likeness of humanity"). Though fully God, Christ chose to operate within human limitations, completely submitting to the Father's will—utter dependence.

Before Jesus begins his ministry, he first faces temptation. Why? Of course, He is perfect, so why go through the charades of being "tempted"? Here's the thing: "It is important to note that Jesus faced the enemy as man, not the Son of God."[7] He didn't stop being God, but He intentionally lived within the limits of humanity. This act shows us that dependence isn't weakness, and it isn't bondage. **Dependence is an essential part of the embodied Christian life.**

We get uncomfortable with this idea, and we must ask ourselves why. We have viewed independence as a strength. I am going to challenge that. Teaching ourselves that we can (and should) do things

7 Warren W. Wiersbe, *The Bible Exposition Commentary* (Wheaton, IL: Victor Books, 1989), 18.

on our own hasn't led to the fullness of life. I would argue it has contributed to our anxiety, our lack of self-worth, and our feeling that we are alone.

Dependence on Each Other

Another theme of the secular worldview that sneaks into our view of our bodies is the emphasis on the individual apart from others. The idea is that what you believe and do is only about what you want. This view is similar to the first, but it is slightly different in that we are both made to be dependent on God, but we are also created to depend on others.

Without this framework of how we are made to be in connection with others, we will continue to struggle with insecurity. We cannot find our confidence by focusing more on ourselves, as secular solutions to body image might suggest. Some secular approaches to body image suggest that instead of our bodies being an ornament (aesthetics) for others, they should be an instrument (purpose) for ourselves.[8] This shift is in a positive direction, but it is incomplete.

It still centers our bodies around personal gratification and self-focus. If we are going to fix our eyes on Jesus to rebuild our body image, then we must also remember that Jesus didn't treat His body as something to preserve or to secure an easy life. He bore unimaginable suffering for our sake, allowing Himself to be spat on, stripped naked, and struck over and over. The world tells us our bodies exist for our own gratification, but Jesus shows us something radically different. Our bodies are not ornaments or instruments for personal fulfillment. Instead, this is the image He gives us: bread, broken; wine, poured out. His body—a living sacrifice. And He calls us to live the same way.

We have been called to offer our bodies as a living sacrifice.

If we only view our bodies as tools for our own benefit, we miss the deeper calling to offer our bodies as living sacrifices, as Scripture

---

8 Lexie Kite and Lindsay Kite, *More Than a Body: Your Body Is an Instrument, Not an Ornament* (Boston: Houghton Mifflin Harcourt, 2021).

teaches. The Gospel pushes us beyond self-focus, reminding us that our bodies are not just for our use but for His glory and the kind of love that gives itself away. Without this shift in focus, we will remain stuck in the same insecurities we are trying to escape.

The more we insist our bodies serve ourselves, the more we distort the image of Christ that we were intended to display. Remember, this kingdom invites us to an upside-down life where we love our enemies (Matthew 5:44), go the extra mile (Matthew 5:41), and deny ourselves (Matthew 16:24) to bring glory to the One we image.

Please don't hear me say what I am not saying. Shifting our focus away from secular definitions of health is not a reason to neglect caring for yourself. It is quite the opposite. We must take care of our bodies because others depend on us to do so. It is a high calling; therefore, your body has a high purpose (more on this to come).

Culture tells us our bodies are meant to serve us. But Scripture calls us to something far more beautiful—a life where we serve the kingdom with our whole selves. The second is far more meaningful, fulfilling, and aligned with what you were made for.

Physical & Spiritual Integration

In *Love Thy Body*, Nancy Pearcey explains that our modern, secular culture has divided the human body into two distinct halves. The first half consists of the *factual*, physical aspects that can be studied scientifically. This scientific realm is where much of the health and fitness industry operates. The second half involves the *value* attributed to those physical aspects.[9] This division significantly affects how we view various issues related to human life. Regarding body image, the ramifications of this separation are this: while your body is composed of matter and can be objectively studied with data, the value is subjective. In other words, you interpret your value based on your feelings. This perspective sharply contrasts with biblical truth.

---

9 Nancy R. Pearcey, *Love Thy Body: Answering Hard Questions about Life and Sexuality* (Grand Rapids, MI: Baker Books, 2018), 42.

It is common for women to find their value in their bodies based on aesthetics. "Look good, feel good," right? Labeling your body as healthy/unhealthy, worthy/unworthy, beautiful/ugly, good/bad, etc., based on how your body appears is all subjective. We have even seen this change across generations and cultures. What is aesthetically "good" has changed.

Or perhaps the body has more value based on how it performs? Again, what is fast, strong, flexible, or fit is subjective, depending on who defines the standards.

This subjectivity is problematic. We are basing how we feel about our bodies on a moving target that has nothing to do with reality.

If looking "good" and feeling "good" are the aims of our body image, beauty, and health pursuits, how do we define good?

God IS good. It is a part of His very nature. Everything He does is good because He cannot contradict His nature. As Ruth Chou Simons writes, "God's goodness isn't simply that He is nice, kind, or helpful; God's goodness is the nonnegotiable standard of beauty, virtue, and wholesomeness that He embodies."[10] Everything God originally made is also good (Genesis 1:32, 1 Timothy 4:4). The definition of good in Genesis from the *Blue Letter Bible* lists adjectives like pleasant, agreeable, excellent, rich, right, and my favorite, **valuable in estimation.**[11]

Your value from a Christian perspective is assigned by your Creator. He has declared His creation good; therefore, your body is good.

This is objectively true. If the human body were insignificant or detestable, we would not have the incarnation. Jesus's entire earthly life and resurrection affirm that our bodies are a good part of creation. While we may know this, the separation of facts and value in our day-to-day lives means we often disconnect the physical

---

10 Ruth Chou Simons, *Pilgrim: 25 Ways God's Character Leads Us Onward* (Nashville: Harvest House Publishers, 2023), 117.

11 "H2896 - tôb - Strong's Hebrew Lexicon (Blue Letter Bible)," *Blue Letter Bible*, accessed May 9, 2025, https://www.blueletterbible.org/lexicon/h2896/kjv/wlc/0-1/.

from the spiritual. We pursue making our bodies "good" through the things we can test and measure.

We keep our bodies squarely in the physical box and place our value in the spiritual. This separation explains why so many Christian women can understand their value as image bearers, and they can still hate their bodies. We rehearse this separation whenever we think what we do with our bodies does not have spiritual implications. The more we rehearse separating these things from one another, the more we unknowingly adopt the mindset of skeptics and materialists. We start to value only the things we can perceive with our five senses, losing the ability to recognize the unseen spiritual realities.

This also explains why we have a hard time integrating Jesus's instructions from His Sermon on the Mount into our lives. We have made our hunger and thirst only spiritual, our self-denial … all spiritual. What we do is spiritual, but we have let our lives in our bodies be formed by a different worldview. And in doing so, we've forgotten: our bodies aren't just recipients of spiritual truth, they're part of how we learn it. This has fractured our spiritual lives from our physical lives—our spiritual and physical formation guided by two opposing belief systems.

How do we reconnect these pieces? Jesus calls us to something so utterly simple yet deeply transformative: "Seek first the kingdom of God" (Matthew 6:33). Not only are we invited to live in this upside-down, set-apart kingdom, but we're also called to *pursue* it. This is the aim, the orientation, the lens through which everything else begins to make sense.

John Stott says it like this, "If we are Christians, everything we do, however 'secular' it may seem (like shopping, cooking, totting up figures in the office, etc.) is 'religious' in the sense that it is done in God's presence and according to God's will."[12]

There is no divide between spiritual and physical, between facts and values, or between what is secular and sacred. God is at the center of it all. And that—right there—is one of the clearest ways

12 John R. W. Stott, *The Message of the Sermon on the Mount* (Downers Grove, IL: InterVarsity Press, 1978), 153.

to uncover the underlying worldview. The line between truth and distortion becomes clear when you consider who is at the center.

The secular worldview always points to the self as the solution, while the biblical worldview always points to Jesus.

Although, by God's grace, I was able to care for my body with better strategies after receiving the news that I was putting my future dreams at risk; I wasn't able to fix the way I felt about myself. It would be a decade before I realized that there wasn't a new book, program, or approach to health and fitness that would help me feel at home in my body.

Instead, the journey to a healthier relationship with my body would begin with a shift in perspective. It starts with recognizing the influence of secular worldviews, embracing the biblical truth of our inherent value as God's creation, and understanding that our bodies are not merely tools for our own use but instruments for His glory. God's goodness extends to our bodies because they reflect His nature and intentions for His good creation. This understanding is vital for a whole and holy view of our bodies where value isn't achieved through appearance, but received through the goodness of God.

If we want to live like our bodies are good, we have to be honest about what's been forming us. The Gospel isn't just something we believe—it's a truth we embody. And it will take unlearning some very loud lies before we can live what we know is true.

The Heart of It

Christ Connection: We were made with limitations to be dependent on God. Jesus didn't live above the human experience—He lived within it. Dependence isn't weakness; it's part of the embodied Christian life.

Community Connection: Our bodies were never meant to serve only ourselves. Jesus didn't treat His body as something for self-preservation or personal comfort—He offered it. In the same way, we are called to offer our bodies as living sacrifices.

Whole Body Connection: We've separated the spiritual and the physical without realizing it. Our bodies are good because God declared them good. They are part of how we live our faith in the world.

3

A Beautiful Body

What do we really want for our bodies?

Beauty is the radiance of the true and the
good, and it is what attracts us to both.

—Stratford Caldecott, *Beauty for Truth's Sake*

I have two core memories from my time working at a weight-loss center, which planted a question in my mind about the sanity of the industry.

I was the newbie, still trying to wrap my brain around the culture. It differed from the one at the fitness center where I also worked. There was no hiding behind the guise of getting stronger and healthier. The agenda is impossible to miss.

The public area of the weight-loss center was small and filled with cubicles where we did our "nutrition" counseling. At the back of the office space was the centerpiece—the scale. On this particular day, a client walked in, skipping pleasantries, and made her way to the back of the office towards the main event of every client check-in. This scale was the kind you see in every doctor's office. The kind that demands stillness while the nurse slides the weights back and forth, determining your worth in pounds. *Is it just me, or are these the worst?*

In a ritual I had come to expect, the woman kicked off her shoes to shave off every extra ounce. I waited for the familiar *thump-thump* of feet on the metal platform, but it was a longer than usual pause. I swiveled in my chair to see what was causing the delay. I glanced over and froze. She was kicking off her pants…

I scanned the room to process what was happening as she removed her pants in front of everyone. I looked around, expecting someone to react, to acknowledge how bizarre this was. No one seemed to bat an eye because when a smaller number is what you want the most, then none of it is really all that surprising.

There was no denying it. These programs prioritize results over care. Friends would do similar programs, get rapid results, and I would experience my own nagging, hidden desire tucked away in my heart. I might not have been as open about this as the woman in the weight-loss center, but the thoughts have always been there in the background. The same endless cycle. The same silent agreement: *this is just what we do.*

These experiences have always made me wonder why we care so much. I've spent years studying the connection between embodiment, spiritual formation, and health. But one element always seemed left out of the conversation: the pervasive influence of our culture's definition of beauty. It's the metaphorical elephant in the room in the health industry. At the time I am writing this, in 2025, the U.S. weight loss market is valued at $90 billion[13], and the global beauty industry is projected to reach $580 billion by 2027.[14] These statistics tell a story: we want to be thinner, and we're afraid of looking older.

Those numbers reflect what the marketing world calls a felt need. Felt needs are what consumers desire. They're what they perceive will make them happier or have a better life. These numbers tell us everything we need to know about what we want. Which of these programs would sell better: "Lose 10 lbs in 30 Days" or "30 Workouts to Help You Live Fuller"?

The answer is evident if you pay attention to what sells. We're not primarily buying *health*; we're buying the promise of a more beautiful version of ourselves. And it reveals an uncomfortable truth: what

---

13 MarketResearch.com, "U.S. Weight Loss Industry Grows to $90 Billion, Fueled by Obesity Drugs Demand," *MarketResearch.com*, April 10, 2023, https://blog.marketresearch.com/u.s.-weight-loss-industry-grows-to-90-billion-fueled-by-obesity-drugs-demand.

14 McKinsey & Company, "The Beauty Market in 2023: A Special State of Fashion Report," *McKinsey & Company*, May 4, 2023, https://www.mckinsey.com/industries/retail/our-insights/the-beauty-market-in-2023-a-special-state-of-fashion-report

we're so often sold as "health" is a distorted version of beauty, and we keep buying it.

What is beauty, and how are we supposed to view it as Christians?

Beauty draws your attention. It makes you pause, sparks awe and wonder, and causes us to worship. We see beauty in the symmetry of shapes, the harmony of notes, and the colors that catch our eyes. We easily see glimpses of beauty in nature: a sunset, an old oak, the coral reef, or a little hummingbird right in our backyard. But we also see beauty in the things we create, such as architecture, literature, music, and art. It is all around us; we were designed to enjoy and recreate it. In this way, beauty is right at home in the Christian worldview, and our desire for it is innate.

Beauty is the fingerprint of our Creator on His design.

Beauty isn't the culprit here, but the twisting of it is. If we want to uncover what the beauty industry is really selling, then we just have to look to the object of worship—the self. We have already concluded that a secular worldview will almost always point us to the self. We have commodified beauty, and we have crafted our bodies into images reflecting a multi-billion-dollar industry instead of into the image of God—*Imago Dei*.

Rooted in Beauty

We often hear the phrase, "Beauty is in the eye of the beholder," implying that beauty is subjective. But in the Christian worldview, beauty isn't subjective at all. We call beautiful what God calls beautiful. We call good what He calls good. We love what He loves, and we seek to follow what He is calling us to do. All true beauty finds its source in the Creator.

Jesus Himself points us to the natural world to illustrate this very point. In the Sermon on the Mount, He tells His disciples to "Observe how the wildflowers of the field grow" (Matthew 6:28). He compares them to Solomon in all his splendor, highlighting that even Solomon's magnificent adornment pales in comparison to the natural beauty of these wildflowers. What is Jesus emphasizing?

> Observe how the wildflowers of the field grow: They don't labor or spin thread. Yet I tell you that not even Solomon in all his splendor was adorned like one of these.
>
> — Matthew 6:28-29

He is, first and foremost, ensuring that He cares for our basic needs like food and clothing. But He is also drawing a parallel to beauty. More specifically, he is talking about "splendor," which can also be translated as glory, majesty, or a thing belonging to Christ. The wildflowers are beautiful *because* He made them. Their beauty is inherent in their design; they don't need to toil or spin to earn or enhance it. They simply *are*. Their existence declares God's glory. Their beauty is a reflection of the One who made them.

This inherent beauty, this reflection of God's glory, is what we see in Christ Himself. The Gospel writers didn't focus on His physical appearance; they focused on His words, His actions, and His very being, defined by His perfect relationship with the Father.

Here's the rub with the beauty of Christ: it has absolutely nothing to do with appearance or aesthetics. In fact, Isaiah 53:2 makes this crystal clear: "He had no form or splendor that we should look at Him, no appearance that we should desire Him."

While cultural beauty standards constantly evolve—our eyebrows, fashion trends, even how we part our hair—biblical beauty remains constant. Specific body shapes may come into fashion, but if we define beauty through the Bible's lens, it always draws our eyes to Christ. In this way, beauty becomes objective. As discussed in the previous chapter, a beautiful body depends on Christ, realizes life through community, and embodies God's goodness.

I'm not saying that expressing creativity through makeup, hairstyles, or fashion is bad. I love these things. I'm a girly girl through and through. The key distinction is between creative expression and sculpting an image to be worshiped for its beauty. If the things that matter most are those that allow others to see Christ in us, we must also be willing to say what doesn't matter. We cannot claim to live differently from the world while still doing everything to blend in with it. We must be willing to ask whose definition of beauty we are pursuing. Are we carving ourselves into idols to be worshiped, or are we allowing God to make us into something of beauty so others will worship Him?

Transformation for the believer always begins in the heart. While the concept of "inner beauty" isn't unique to Christianity, there's a significant difference. The problem with looking inward for beauty apart from Christ is that we know our flaws. This awareness often leads to insecurity. We want to display our value, worth, and beauty, but deep down, we know we'll never measure up.

Insecurity and self-absorption are two sides of the same coin: both cause us to think more of ourselves, amplifying our feelings of inadequacy. The way out of that spiral isn't found in thinking less of ourselves or more of ourselves; it's found in thinking rightly about ourselves through Christ. The Christian life is a confident one when we understand where our confidence comes from—where our beauty comes from.

Jesus came as both fully man and fully God, showing what it means to live fully human in perfect union with God. Through the empowering work of the Holy Spirit, our will, our emotions, and our desires can be beautifully ordered and submitted to the Father's will. **The inside job of beauty must be a work of the Holy Spirit through Christ.**

When we try to beautify ourselves from the outside in, we create idols of ourselves. We will always feel inadequate when we attempt to create beauty from the inside out in our strength. Both approaches lead only to more insecurity. Both approaches rely on subjective beauty defined by whichever way the cultural wind blows. In contrast, objective beauty is grounded in the Holy Spirit's work within us, providing a stable foundation we can always rely on. This objective beauty points us away from self and towards Christ, inviting us to reflect His image in a way that brings true confidence.

Reflecting Beauty

Even while immersed in studying and writing about God's purpose for our bodies, I recently found myself slipping back into a familiar conversation with a group of Christian women about how our bodies seem to fall short. One woman lamented about her post-baby body, another about struggles to see the scale move, and I, without even thinking, chimed in with my own insecurities. It was a sobering moment. Even as we professed to believe that our worth is found in Christ, we were tearing ourselves down, perpetuating the same messages the world feeds us.

It is socially acceptable for women to objectify their own bodies, bonding over their insecurities, comparing weights, and lamenting over frustrations with bodies that refuse to comply. But when we grumble about the appearance of our bodies, there are spiritual/communal consequences. Communally, we perpetuate the objectification of women. How can we, in one breath, be outraged by the unrealistic ideals placed on women's bodies and, in the other breath, lead the charge of the war on our own bodies?

We echo the world's values every time we elevate appearance above identity. Complaining about how we look reveals how deeply the world is shaping us. We model the world's message when we focus on what our bodies *are not* instead of glorifying God for what they *are*. We inadvertently reinforce ideals about our bodies that damage the body of Christ.

Jesus modeled and called us to something radically different: love. "By this everyone will know that you are my disciples, if you love one another" (John 13:35 CSB). This love isn't merely a spiritual idea; it's practical. It's a way of being in the world and seeing others and ourselves through God's eyes. Natasha Crain's distinction between secular and Godly love is helpful here: "Secular love often means wanting for others what they want for themselves. Godly love means wanting for others what God wants for them—even when that's not what they currently desire."[15]

Therefore, we should encourage one another in ways that glorify God, not ourselves. When we objectify or complain about the bodies He has given us— bodies given by our Creator to experience life, serve the world, and share the good news, we diminish His good creation and wound the body

> So if one member suffers, all the members suffer with it; if one member is honored, all the members rejoice with it.
>
> —1 Corinthians 12:26

of Christ. We are all part of that body, intricately connected. When one part suffers, we all suffer (1 Corinthians 12:26). Our words, our attitudes, and our actions toward our bodies have ripple effects within the community of faith.

Our collective approach to our bodies, motivated by love for God and love for our neighbors, extends to our whole selves. It speaks volumes about what we value. When love drives our conversations and actions rather than complaint or self-obsession, we honor the Creator and make Christ visible to the world. In a culture defined by insecurity and comparison, we can choose to stand apart, embracing our bodies as intentional creations of God and living out His love through them.

Embodying Beauty

Christ is always the best measure for us; however, we can learn from the lives of women in the Bible. The Old Testament has an interesting pattern regarding beauty, and it is worth noticing because it makes what we see in the Gospels even more astounding.

---

15 Natasha Crain, *Talking with Your Kids about Jesus: 30 Conversations Every Christian Parent Must Have* (Minneapolis: Bethany House, 2020), 155.

Throughout the Old Testament, there's a recurring emphasis on physical beauty regarding women. Sarai (later Sarah), Abram's wife, is described as "beautiful" (Genesis 12:11, 20:2). She was so striking that Abram feared for his life, convinced her beauty would put him in danger. This attention to beauty isn't incidental. It's a thread woven through these stories, often revealing how women were seen.

Rachel, known for her captivating beauty, became one of Jacob's wives (Genesis 29:17).

Abigail, described as beautiful and intelligent, became David's wife after demonstrating wisdom and courage (1 Samuel 25:3).

Tamar's beauty tragically led to a devastating assault by her half-brother Amnon (2 Samuel 13:1).

And Esther, through what was essentially a beauty contest, was chosen to become queen of Persia (Esther 2:7).

In each of these instances, physical attractiveness is a key characteristic highlighted in their introductions, often playing a significant role in the unfolding events of their lives.

This recurring emphasis on physical beauty is not a commentary on the women but on the cultural values of that time. Physical appearance was closely tied to status and worth in many ancient societies. A beautiful woman was seen as a valuable asset, and her beauty could influence her family's social standing or political alliances. These descriptions, therefore, are not simply neutral observations; they reveal the priorities of the culture in which these stories were written. Would we say our culture is all that different?

But then we turn to the Gospels; it's as if a light suddenly shines in a dark room. The lens shifts. The criteria change. Where the Old Testament often highlights physical beauty, the Gospels offer a radically different perspective. Jesus values something different from the culture. We see women described not by their outward appearance but by their *inward* qualities of devotion, faithfulness, sacrifice, and courage. And yet, many of these women would have been considered *undesirable* by the standards of their time.

Think about Mary, the mother of Jesus. We're told she was a virgin (important for the fulfillment of the prophecy), and that she found favor with God, chosen for a sacred role in His redemptive plan (Luke 1:26–31). There's no mention of her physical appearance. Instead, we see her obedience to a costly calling (Luke 1:38).

Mary Magdalene is remembered for her unwavering devotion to Jesus, even at the foot of the cross (John 19:25; Mark 15:47).

The Samaritan woman at the well (John 4), an outcast in her community, is transformed by her encounter with Jesus and becomes a messenger of good news.

The woman healed of bleeding (Mark 5:25-34), likely considered ritually unclean and marginalized, is commended for her extraordinary faith.

Martha and Mary of Bethany (Luke 10:38-42) are contrasted not by their looks but by their different expressions of love and service to Jesus.

The "sinful woman" who anointed Jesus's feet (Luke 7:37-38) is remembered for her profound humility and extravagant worship—a stark contrast to the judgment she likely faced from others.

Over and over again, the New Testament portrays women who through qualities such as faith, humility, devotion, sacrifice, and obedience, glorify God through their bodies. Mary's pregnancy, the demons cast out of bodies, the bleeding body that was healed, the proclaiming of God's truth to her town, the sitting with, the worshiping … all done in bodies, leaving an eternal legacy.

The women in the Gospels were beautiful because they glorified God as they were made to—with their bodies, in their stories, and through their surrender.

Have you ever seen a woman who quietly tends to those around her, noticing what others overlook? She serves with humility and care. Or the woman who can make an ordinary meal extraordinary with creativity and generosity? She hosts with love. Or the woman who explains something so clearly, so thoughtfully, that you see the world differently because of it? She teaches with wisdom.

We experience deep fulfillment when we find a place to use our God-given, individual gifts to bless the people we care about because it brings harmony and balance to the world. Your gifts bring beauty to the body of Christ.

As we slowly unravel these ideas about beauty from the secular worldview and piece them back together, we get a brand-new desire for our bodies. This shift calls us not only to change what we *believe*, but it calls us to something even more challenging … to change what we *want*. It requires examining the desires and insecurities we've tucked away, forcing us to finally declare: *We want Jesus more than anything else.* The commitment to seek His kingdom first allows us to live lives that are fully cohesive with what we believe. We no longer have to feel like we are seeking the world's answers for our bodies while simultaneously seeking God's wisdom for our spirits. When our heart's desires align with our beliefs, we move closer to creating a vision for a wholeness set apart for a holy calling.

My last memory from that job at the weight loss center happened just a few months after the weigh-in incident.

A mother and daughter sat across from me, sliding their food logs across the desk. Week after week, they recorded every bite and every sip, following the program to perfection—1,200 calories a day of shakes, bars, and frozen meals. They had lost some weight, but now? They were stuck. Their bodies had hit a plateau, and there was nowhere left to go. Because when you're already at 1,200 calories, what is left to cut?

That's when it hit me: I had wanted to help women feel better in their bodies, but I was feeding the very dissatisfaction I longed to free them from. The same dissatisfaction I longed to free myself from. I couldn't do it anymore. So I quit.

I think about those women often. I wonder if they're still on the weight-loss hamster wheel, or if they've realized the number on the scale was never a measure of what made them beautiful.

The war against the body never ends unless we choose to stop playing by the culture's rules of erasing pounds and years.

What we want isn't a smaller number or fewer wrinkles. It's knowing that our bodies matter, that they are good, and that they were made for more.

And we only find that kind of clarity when we begin to understand the body's purpose—our purpose.

The Heart of It

Christ Connection: We are called to reflect the beauty of Christ, whose splendor had nothing to do with appearance and everything to do with obedience, sacrifice, and love—made visible through the work of the Holy Spirit in us.

Community Connection: The way we speak about our bodies— especially in front of one another—shapes more than our self-perception; it shapes the body of Christ, reinforcing or resisting the cultural messages we claim to reject.

Whole Body Connection: True beauty is not subjective or shifting; it's the natural result of a life that glorifies God.

4

The Purpose of the Body

Why do we have bodies?

What would it mean to believe the Gospel,
not just in my brain, but also in my body?

—Tish Harrison Warren, *Liturgy of the Ordinary*

This book was going to have all the answers.

Every month or so, I grab a mainstream health book. It's usually the one everyone on the internet says is life changing. I love knowing which way the wind is blowing in the health and fitness industry, and I am always trying to take better care of myself and my family. If there is promising research out there, I want to read it!

The human body is fascinating. I enjoy science and research because I believe with every fiber of my being that they reveal God's handiwork. Just like some people see a sunset, mountains, or a beautiful flower and experience the breathtaking awe of God's design, I experience the same sentiment when glimpsing into the intricacies of the human body.

After listening to the author being interviewed on a podcast, I wasted no seconds ordering a newly released book. I was nodding my head along with everything she was saying. She gets it! Finally, a health book that wasn't so niched down that it was totally irrelevant. I had felt like the gist of every health book was this: *The secret to revolutionizing your health is in this one single solution.* These books fill the shelves at used bookstores because, it turns out, they never solve our actual problem.

Thank goodness Amazon delivered next day because this book would be different from all the others. With my no-bleed, gel highlighter in hand, I dove into the book, and about halfway through this particular *New York Times* best seller, I got a familiar feeling in the pit of my stomach. Fear. All the bites of food, exposure to toxins, our drinking water, polluted air, lack of proper breathing, and screens. There was no time to sit and read the book because there was so much I needed to do that I wasn't currently doing. I was no longer a girl cozied up with a brand-new book. Instead, I was a mom overwhelmed and near panic. There was just so much to … control.

The theory of evolution has deeply influenced how we view our bodies. More specifically, it has influenced the way we define the **purpose** of our bodies. What meaning can we attribute to our existence if we were not created?

Darwin's ideas have subtly shaped our understanding of ourselves and how we pursue the care of our bodies. If you've read a scientifically grounded book on health, chances are it's rooted in assumptions that stem from evolutionary theory. Whether you realize it or not, these ideas seep into the waters we swim in every day. We don't even notice them.

So what is the purpose of the body if evolutionary theory is the foundation on which we are building our health practices? *Survival.* Once you see it, you won't be able to unsee it. Read almost any book on health, strip away all the industry jargon and data, and it is essentially an attempt to escape death for as long as possible using human will. I just googled the best-selling health books, and here are some current titles that popped up at the top: *Outlive, How Not to Die, Lifespan, Can't Hurt Me: Master Your Mind and Defy the Odds.* These titles were just in the current top ten. The messaging is not so subtly there: your survival depends on getting it all right.

I'm not saying these books are bad. In fact, one is on my own wish list to read. But we need to recognize that it's never just information. The messages tell a story. And it's one that is at odds with the one true story we long for. A *better* story.

No wonder women feel so much stress, fear, and overwhelm when trying to make "healthy choices." We have been listening to voices that tell us our goal is to survive, avoid death, and that we are the ones in control of it all. Do you see how this is at odds with the Gospel?

I finished the last page of the book with a single, unexpected thought. *Where is the hope in this?*

But as Christians, our bodies are not a product of survival of the fittest but are created for a divine purpose.

Presence

"Inconceivable!"

I recently rewatched The Princess Bride with my two boys. Let's just say the sword fighting and silliness weren't quite enough to distract them from the fact that, in the end, it's still a love story. Still, when Inigo Montoya utters the words, "You keep using that word; I do not think it means what you think it means," I laugh because he finally said what we were all thinking!

Similarly, within Christian circles, the phrase "Your body is a temple" has become somewhat of a catchphrase—a spiritual equivalent to Vizzini's misuse of the word 'inconceivable.' While it sounds profound to say it, it has been misapplied to go on a mission to beautify, strengthen, or enhance our outer self. This is how workouts and weight loss have gotten intermixed with this piece of Scripture. The temple's purpose was to have a place for God to meet with His people. It has nothing to do with fitness.

We must finish the sentence that is being quoted from Paul in 1 Corinthians 6:19, "Don't you know that your body is the temple **of the Holy Spirit** who is in

> Don't you know that your body is a temple of the Holy Spirit who is in you, whom you have from God? You are not your own, for you were bought with a price. So glorify God with your body.
>
> —1 Corinthians 6:19-20

you, whom you have from God? *You are not your own*, for you were bought with a price." (emphasis mine).

He's not talking about fitness. He's writing to a church entangled in sexual sin, calling them to holiness, and to live lives that reflect the presence of God. Not appearance. *Presence.*

The purpose of the body, then, is to be submitted to the work of the Holy Spirit so that when others encounter us, they encounter Christ.

This is big and worth repeating. The purpose of the body is that when others **encounter us**, they experience something of His presence. God chose to reveal Himself by the power of the Holy Spirit through His disciples. That's us in this generation.

In breaking down some major differences between the secular and biblical worldviews, we touched on the theological idea of kenosis—how Christ, in taking on human flesh, showed us that our limits are not flaws to be overcome but reminders of our dependence on the Father. When we embrace our limits, we don't hide Christ— we reflect Him.

As Christ entered the wilderness, each Gospel describes Him in slightly different terms, but they all point to the same reality: He was led, driven, and filled by the Spirit of God. Matthew tells us He was **led** (*anagō*, Matthew 4:1); Mark says He was **driven out** (*ekballō*, Mark 1:12); and Luke describes Him as **full** (*plērēs*, Luke 4:1) of the Holy Spirit. These words may differ, but the picture is unified: Jesus, though fully God, lived in perfect surrender to the Spirit.[16]

And here's the miracle—we are filled with that same Spirit— not because we've earned it or reached some physical or spiritual benchmark, but because we believe. This is how we reflect God in the world—not through striving but through surrender. *This* is what it means to say that our bodies are temples of the Holy Spirit.

We cannot twist these verses about our bodies being a temple with marketing for health and fitness programs. If we were to play

16 *Blue Letter Bible*, "Matthew 4 – Greek Lexicon," https://www.blueletterbible.org/csb/mat/4/1/t_conc_933001; *Blue Letter Bible*, "Mark 1 – Greek Lexicon," https://www.blueletterbible.org/csb/mar/1/12/t_conc_958012; *Blue Letter Bible*, "Luke 4 – Greek Lexicon," https://www.blueletterbible.org/csb/luk/4/1/t_conc_977001.

this out to its logical conclusion, then sick bodies, disabled bodies, old bodies, etc., would be less-than-temples for the Holy Spirit. I don't see evidence of that in the Scriptures. It's often the opposite.

The problem with using Scripture to support secular culture (i.e. lift weights because your body is a temple) is that we end up with these sneaky little subconscious lies. It's the lie that the body is a project to manage, a thing to perfect, a commodity to control. The following line says: "You are not your own, for you were bought at a price. So glorify God with your body" (1 Corinthians 6:19–20).

I have justified health and fitness as a good and God-glorifying endeavor by misapplying these Scriptures when I was justifying an idol in my life. The reflection of Christ oftentimes doesn't look like what the world would elevate as an image of health.

For example, a newly postpartum mom practicing stillness with her littles shows the presence of the Holy Spirit. The grandma who exudes joy and peace even in the middle of a life-changing diagnosis reminds us that Christ has defeated death. The woman who embraces gratitude and worship in relationship to her food, regardless of a number on a scale, reminds us we are not of this world. They show us these things with their bodies. We glimpse God's goodness here on earth.

Relationship

In the Western world, we tend to think of identity as individual and self-contained. But Scripture paints a different picture—one of deep, interconnected belonging. Paula Gooder writes, "One of the reasons why Christianity struggles to find a home in the Western world is because Christianity is underpinned by an understanding of corporate identity, in which who you really are can only be understood together rather than apart."[17]

In the same way that the words "our body is a temple" can become a cliche and lose their depth of meaning, the words "the

---

17 Paula Gooder, *Body: Biblical Spirituality for the Whole Person* (London: SPCK, 2016), 109.

body" referring to the church can be lost on us. However, how we serve one another, how we speak to each other, how we resolve conflict, and how we care for our families should give the world a glimpse into the spiritual truths about the kingdom of God. It puts flesh on the unseen spiritual realities.

If we were never meant to live alone, then it is through relationships with others that we are formed. Not just socially, but spiritually. Through the ordinary acts of showing up, listening, serving, and being served, we are becoming who we were always meant to be.

I love the story Kelly M. Kapic shares in his book *You're Only Human*, where a professor has his class introduce themselves with one key catch—they cannot reference any groups they are a part of in their intro. The challenge begins from the moment they state their name, which would tie them to their family ... community.[18]

Try it.

My name is Ashley, which is a name chosen for me before I was born, and it ties me to my family's story. As a mom of two boys and a wife, I live out roles that are relational at their core. Homeschooling my kids ties me to a broader network of families pursuing the same goals. Even writing opens a conversation with an audience, shaped by the voices and feedback of a community. The Bible study group that I'm a part of connects me with people who gather to study alongside me. I earned a degree in health studies, a pursuit guided by professors, classmates, and the shared experience of a college community. Even hobbies such as reading connect me to the ideas, stories, and perspectives of others. Each facet of my life ties me to people—to community.

We are not designed to be self-contained beings; we are image-bearers, made for relationship with God and with one another. And since our bodies are how we engage with and relate to people, it is also a part of shaping who we become.

---

18 Kelly M. Kapic, *You're Only Human: How Your Limits Reflect God's Design and Why That's Good News* (Grand Rapids, MI: Brazos Press, 2022), 76–78.

Our bodies give birth and hold hands with loved ones. They offer hugs for comfort and play—pushing toddlers in swings at the park, dancing with our spouses in the kitchen, and laughing with friends until our sides ache. Our bodies communicate through touch, gestures, expressions, and words. If identity is shaped within community, then it is through the body that we become who we are.

Science affirms what Scripture has long told us. A Harvard study spanning 85 years found that the best predictor of health isn't diet or exercise, but relationships.[19] This surprising conclusion highlights what we instinctively know: taking care of our bodies is vital, but the richness of life and our well-being depend on the strength of our connections.

This is why understanding the purpose of our bodies must include how they are designed for relationships. God Himself exists in perfect relationship—Father, Son, and Holy Spirit—and He created us in His image to reflect that relational nature.

Our bodies serve a greater purpose than mere survival. God formed them for relationships.

Purpose

I have more books than I can count that try to answer the question of who we are. It's a question as old as humanity itself. Something in us longs to know our place. Not just generally as people, but personally. You and me. Specifically. We've named that, as believers, our sense of meaning is rooted in Christ and shaped in community. But what does that mean for us as individuals? What does it mean to live in our particular bodies with our particular stories?

You are not just a random assignment of DNA. God created you both body and soul as a whole person, designed to live out His purposes through your embodied life. God's Word declares it so, but you can also see this in the very life of Christ.

19 Liz Mineo, "Over Nearly 80 Years, Harvard Study Has Been Showing How to Live a Healthy and Happy Life," *Harvard Gazette*, April 11, 2017, https://news.harvard.edu/gazette/story/2017/04/over-nearly-80-years-harvard-study-has-been-showing-how-to-live-a-healthy-and-happy-life/.

Jesus was born in a particular body for a specific purpose.

Everything about Jesus was specific and intentional: His gender, His heritage, His parents, the location of His birth, and even the timeline of His entrance into the world. These details were not arbitrary; they were essential to fulfilling God's plan.

We can see this up close through the genealogy found in Matthew. Genealogies were critical in Jewish culture. They determined land allotments and who served in the priesthood, and they were also essential in identifying the Messiah.

Matthew's Gospel traces Jesus's lineage:

- through Jacob (Genesis 28:13-15),

- through the tribe of Judah (Genesis 49:8),

- through the family tree of Jesse (Isaiah 11:1),

- and through the branch of David (Jeremiah 23:5).

Every branch of His family tree traces back to Old Testament prophecy.

Most scholars agree that Matthew's genealogy traces Joseph's lineage. However, because of the virgin birth, Jesus wasn't Joseph's biological son. Still, as the firstborn in Joseph's household, Jesus had the legal right to inherit the throne of King David, fulfilling one of the key messianic prophecies. What's especially fascinating is that many scholars believe Luke's genealogy traces Mary's lineage. Matthew's genealogy shows the legal fulfillment of prophecy, while Luke's highlights the biological fulfillment.[20]

There is a whole world to discover within both genealogies in the Gospels, uncovering that no detail about the body Jesus was born into was happenstance.

If we are to hold a biblical view of our bodies, we must understand that every aspect of the body we were born into serves a particular purpose—whether we would choose it for ourselves or not. Our gender, ethnicity, family background, and DNA are not

20 Skip Heitzig, *Bloodline: Tracing God's Rescue Plan from Eden to Eternity* (Colorado Springs: Worthy Publishing, 2018), 150–151.

incidental. They are part of the story God is telling through us. These embodied details locate us in time and place, grounding how we reflect Him in the world.

If this is true, how do we reconcile the brokenness we experience in our bodies because of sin and death with our purpose? We are born with abnormalities, pains, and diseases that bring grief, fear, and hardship. These realities were not part of God's original design in creation—He called the body good. But since the fall, the world, including our bodies, has been marked by brokenness. And yet, even here, God has not abandoned His design. In His goodness, He redeems and purposes every bit of it.

We'll explore the redemption of our broken bodies more deeply in a later chapter, but for now, it's worth saying this clearly: suffering and pain are not what God originally—or ultimately—desires for our bodies. But in His mercy, He can bring good *through* it. And when we surrender our pain to Him, we see glimpses of His redemptive work, even here—in the waiting.

In John 9, the disciples ask Jesus why a man was blind from birth. It is natural to ask why. The underlying assumption is, what did he do wrong to cause this? Jesus's answer is shocking: He was blind so that God's works might be displayed in him. His blindness was not a punishment from God or a consequence of his own sin. His bodily limits had a purpose, ultimately leading to a miraculous display of God's power when Jesus restored his sight.

Just like God's work was displayed in the blind man through the restoration of his sight, we see the ultimate purpose of Jesus's ministry fulfilled by His own bodily suffering. Although Christ remained fully God, He operated within some of humanity's limitations, allowing Himself to be crucified. It is through His literal, physical death that humanity has the opportunity for redemption.

Life through death. Purpose through pain.

We can ask *why* God chooses to work the way He does, but I have learned that this question doesn't give us many answers. What we can ask is *how* God works. One way is through our pain.

C.S. Lewis is famously quoted: "We can ignore even pleasure. But pain insists upon being attended to. God whispers to us in our pleasures, speaks in our conscience, but shouts in our pains: it is his megaphone to rouse a deaf world."[21]

Our pain, our limits, and our brokenness often draw us to the only One who promises hope. Our physical pain reminds us of a spiritual reality that we are living the "now and not yet" life in these bodies. We steward God's good creation, but we also know that it has been affected by the fall. And when we allow God to be glorified through our limits, we draw others to Him. We begin to come full circle—drawing near to Christ, drawing others to Christ, and living out our purpose in these bodies: to glorify God.

If the purpose of our physical body is survival—to keep us alive, then we either do everything in our power to ensure our longevity, or we do nothing because we don't see the point. Either way, it is a bleak picture of what it means to be embodied. But, if we look to the incarnation of Christ, who was born into a specific body for a particular purpose from the moment He was formed in the womb until the moment He laid His life down on the cross, we find that our entire embodied existence has a purpose for the kingdom of God here on earth. Jesus's embodied life reveals the purpose of ours and teaches us that merely surviving is not the same as living a life rooted in eternity.

---

21 C. S. Lewis, *The Problem of Pain* (New York: HarperOne, 2001), 91.

The Heart of It

Christ Connection: The purpose of the body is presence. Just as Christ came in the flesh and was filled with the Spirit, we too are temples—dwelling places of the same Spirit.

Community Connection: We were made to be formed and to flourish through embodied life together. Our bodies are how we show up, serve, and share in the life of Christ with one another.

Whole Body Connection: God didn't give you a generic body. He gave you this one, including its shape, its story, its aches. You were born in your particular body for a particular purpose.

5

A Healthy Body

How should we care for our bodies?

Connection is health.

—Norman Wirzba, *Food and Faith*

Connection is health. I paused as I read the words. I needed to think about that. Could it be that simple? Here I am in my 40s, having spent my entire adult life trying to understand the body, and this seemed so simple yet oddly profound.

I had been surrounded by similar messaging in my work: mind-body connection, holistic health, integrative medicine. Even the software used in the Pilates and barre studios I taught in was called "Mindbody." The language was everywhere, but for me, it always felt hollow—just more buzzwords tied to products or programs, more solutions to a wrongly defined problem.

We've been sold the idea that health is an outcome, a goal to achieve, something you chase. It's beauty. It's longevity. But just because something "works" doesn't make it good, especially when we define good by the reflection of God's nature and intentions through His creation.

What is health from a biblical perspective? Well, Wirzba was on to something. It's connection.

But here is the key: it's not just *random* connection; it must be ordered connection.

Jesus's language is filled with order and prioritization:

- "But seek first the kingdom of God" (Matthew 6:33)

- "Love the Lord your God with all your heart, with all your soul, and with all your mind. This is the greatest and most important command." (Matthew 22:37–38)

- "You hypocrite, first take the plank out of your own eye, and then you will see clearly to remove the speck from your brother's eye." (Matthew 7:5)

- "First, be reconciled to your brother, and then come and offer your gift." (Matthew 5:24)

Scripture repeats this rhythm—first things first. This doesn't mean we have to rigidly check off a list. Connect with God, check. Connect with others, check. Integrate our physical and spiritual selves, check. But it does mean we can't skip these essential connections and expect things to go well for us.

My younger self didn't understand this. I treated every part of my life as a separate category to manage. Spiritual things like church, prayer, and reading Scripture went into one bucket. Taking care of my body went into another. Work, family, and friendships each had their own place. Without realizing it, I rehearsed fragmentation, dividing my life into compartments that never fully connected.

But when we understand ordered connection, everything shifts. Instead of juggling separate pieces, we see our lives as one cohesive, integrated whole where every aspect is aligned under God's design.

When we try to skip ahead, armed only with knowledge of the body, apart from the wisdom and guidance of the One who formed us, it doesn't work. It's like playing a game of whack-a-mole—solving one problem, only for another one to pop up. Then, we become more stressed and less healthy, look for more solutions, and the cycle continues.

Connection to Christ

One of the biggest challenges for Christian women when it comes to health is the weight of responsibility we carry as caretakers. We are the gatekeepers of our homes, and we take that role seriously—and rightly so—it is a good and beautiful calling. We research the safest products, choose the most nourishing foods, monitor habits, and carefully weigh medical decisions for our families. We pour ourselves out, ensuring the well-being of those we love.

But in the midst of all this, it's easy to let our role as caretakers overshadow our connection to the One who sustains us. We convince ourselves that if we work harder, plan better, or find the perfect solution; we can create health and security for those around us.

But Jesus delivers the same message to us over and over again:

- But seek first the kingdom of God (Matthew 6:33)
- I am the Way, the Truth, and the Light (John 14:6)
- Come to Me (Matthew 11:28)
- Abide in Me (John. 15:4)
- Follow Me (Luke 9:23)
- Come after Me (Luke 14:26)

There is an ongoing theme in Jesus's message. His call is always relational, always invitational. Come. Abide. Follow. These words aren't merely about belief—they are about connection, about a life fully oriented toward Him. These aren't just spiritual ideas; they're meant to be lived.

We do not simply make Jesus Lord over certain parts of our lives while white-knuckling control over others—especially when it comes to our health. God is sovereign in every area. The Christian life is not about compartmentalized faith but moment-by-moment faithfulness. When we grasp this, discipline becomes less about control and more about surrender. If our planning and preparation have replaced prayer, we are not walking in faith—we are rehearsing self-sufficiency. We say we trust God but order our lives as if everything depends on us.

If we use habits to gain control over our lives, we will find ourselves exhausted. It's just striving, rebranded. It doesn't matter if we call them habits, rhythms, or goals—these are simply the outworkings of where we have placed our faith. Healthy habits without a heart of surrender to Jesus are just more things to check off the list. And when our faith is in ourselves and our own capabilities, overwhelm is inevitable.

Healthy habits can be daily liturgies of dependence—or subtle rehearsals of self-reliance.

Self-control is listed as a fruit of the Spirit. But there is a difference between trying to control everything in our own strength and relying on the Holy Spirit to produce self-control in us. The former feeds our stress, fueled by self-preservation and self-reliance. The latter leads to rest as we continue to lay down our lives before God.

Discipline in the Christian life is not about rigidly controlling every aspect of our lives. It's about being faithful to what God calls us to, even when it's challenging.

Self-control is not about exerting more willpower—it's about surrender. It's choosing what is good over what is easy.

We must start with surrender. We cannot skip it. Chapter 9 explores surrender more tangibly as we look at how rest becomes one of the clearest ways we live that truth with our bodies. Without surrendering to Christ, we will approach health backward, chasing outcomes instead of living whole.

Connection to Community

When we define health as Christians, we should always consider our bodies within the context of the body of Christ. Research is slowly revealing what God's Word has already declared as the design for humanity. We were never made to live in isolation.

Do a quick Google search of loneliness and mortality, and we find that social isolation is associated with an increased risk of *all-*

cause mortality. Loneliness is associated with a wide range of chronic health conditions, including heart disease, high blood pressure, and cognitive decline.[22] It affects brain function, worsens mental health[23], and has even been shown to reduce life expectancy.[24]

Our connection to other humans affects the entirety of our health. This understanding comes at a critical time in our culture because we live in an era where you can do just about anything from the comfort of the four walls of your home. More access to information has led to less access to other humans ... real humans, in real bodies.

"Technology is not inherently evil, but it tends to become the platform of choice to express the fantasy of human autonomy."[25]

Do you need an answer, a recipe, insight into a problem, or help with home repair? It's all a Google search away. Can these online resources be great tools, and can we connect with people we couldn't have without them? Sure. However, we no longer experience the need for others in a real, tangible way, and it has left the door open for isolation and loneliness to sneak in before we even notice. It's easy to confuse a connection made through a screen with the embodied connection that God designed us for. It's not the same.

It's not the same as looking someone in the eye to see their real-time reaction. It isn't the same as reaching across the table and hugging them when they share devastating news. It isn't the same as hearing the tone in their voice change when they begin to talk

---

22 Emily Harris, "Meta-Analysis: Social Isolation, Loneliness Tied to Higher Mortality," *JAMA* 330, no. 3 (July 18, 2023): 211, https://jamanetwork.com/journals/jama/article-abstract/2806852.

23 A. J. Finley & S. M. Schaefer, "Affective Neuroscience of Loneliness: Potential Mechanisms Underlying the Association Between Perceived Social Isolation, Health, and Well-Being," *Journal of Psychiatry and Brain Science* 7 (2022): e220011, https://doi.org/10.20900/jpbs.20220011.

24 Xuexin Yu et al., "Association of Cumulative Loneliness with All-Cause Mortality among Middle-Aged and Older Adults in the United States, 1996 to 2019," *Proceedings of the National Academy of Sciences* 120, no. 51 (December 11, 2023): e2306819120, https://doi.org/10.1073/pnas.2306819120.

25 Tony Reinke, *12 Ways Your Phone Is Changing You* (Wheaton, IL: Crossway, 2017), 34.

about something they are passionate about. It isn't the same as sitting shoulder-to-shoulder with someone in prayer.

Jesus modeled ordered connection. He withdrew often to be with the Father (Luke 5:16), and from that place of intimacy, He moved toward others by teaching, healing, and investing personally in His disciples. He never rushed connections. As His body, the church, we are called to follow the same pattern.

Connection isn't just good theology—it's good for our health

Whole Body Connection

As a culture, we've come to recognize the importance of whole health—mind, body, and emotions. But long before we had the language for it, Jesus was already pointing us toward true wholeness.

> He said to him, "Love the Lord your God with all your heart, with all your soul, and with all your mind."
>
> — Matthew 22:37

In Matthew 22:37-38 He says, "Love the Lord your God with all your heart, and with all your soul, and with all your mind." Jesus followed this by saying, "This is the greatest and most important command."

This Scripture is interesting because when Jesus implores us to love Him with our whole selves, it implies that we could also do the opposite—loving Him with only parts of ourselves.

What if we redefined our health goals as connection goals? It's hard to put connection on a to-do list. You have to be slow, intentional, and fully present. Haven't we all been craving this? We taste it in the patient work of gardening. In the warmth of a meal made together. In the stillness of reading a book just for the joy of it. We feel it when we make eye contact, sit across from someone, and stay long enough to listen. A retreat from the fractured, hurried way of living we've come to accept as normal.

But so often, we treat our bodies like machines to manage. Quick workouts. Grab-and-go meals. Substitutes that replace what slow care was meant to offer. We have made our bodies something to maintain instead of something to live in that is fundamentally a part of who we are. We treat our bodies as if they are like cars that need to get us from place to place—just needing fuel and regular maintenance checks. Our bodies aren't our whole identity, but we can't separate them from who we are.

There is a temptation in Christian communities to make the spiritual more important than the physical. This will often lead us to conclude that our bodies are less important than our minds, hearts, and souls. We do not see any evidence of this idea in the Gospels. Jesus came in a body, healed bodies, was resurrected in a body, ascended in a body, and remains in a body.

However, the eternal *is* more important than the temporal.[26]

When aligned with the spiritual, the body can be of eternal significance and impact. We are no longer grasping at a purpose, beauty, or health that will ultimately fade and deteriorate. Instead, there is a greater purpose to our choices, sacrifices, and discipline. They no longer strengthen the physical body for a temporary result but deepen our relationships with God, our world, and ourselves.

We have spent the first chapters of this book recognizing that body image is not about fixing our bodies but fixing our minds and hearts on truth. We must filter our ideas about our bodies through a biblical lens so that we can separate true health from cultural beauty standards and live as though our bodies exist for something far greater than temporary self-improvement.

The Gospel vision for health is when everything is connected: our bodies, minds, and souls are all submitted to the authority of Christ and lived out through community with others.

The strategies may vary. These are the specifics of how you carry out the vision. The choices you make depend on your family

---

26 Natasha Crain, *Faithfully Different: Regaining Biblical Clarity in a Secular Culture* (Minneapolis: Bethany House, 2022), 177.

dynamics, your callings, your specific season of life, you and your family's needs, and your personal convictions. But your strategies should align and support the vision.

Now, with a clearer understanding of biblical health, we can map out what it means to care for our bodies in a way that aligns with our vision. We're not just looking for temporary improvement; we're seeking a life that reflects God's design—connected and set apart for the kingdom—a body shaped by the Gospel.

The Heart of It

Christ Connection: Health begins not with striving, but with surrender. When our habits flow from a heart connected to Christ, they become a faithful response to His presence.

Community Connection: We were never meant to pursue health in isolation. Our connection to others isn't optional—it's essential, because embodied presence is central to both our health and our formation.

Whole Body Connection: True health isn't just a collection of habits—it's a way of living where our physical, emotional, and spiritual lives are aligned under the authority of Christ and lived out through real connection.

Part 2
Embodying the Gospel

Having a body is a lot of work.

—Tish Harrison Warren, *Liturgy of the Ordinary*

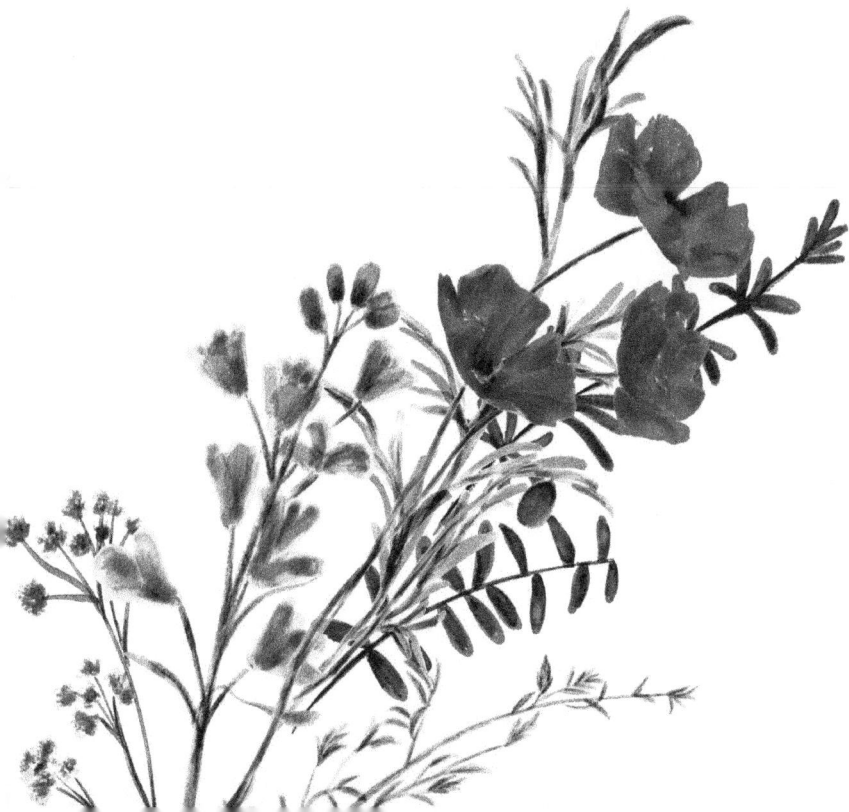

6

Nourishment

How do we align nutrition
with the Gospel vision for health?

We can no more make food grow than we can make rain
fall. We are, as Wendell Berry writes, 'living from mystery,'
dependent on forces we can't control and processes we don't
fully understand. A physical reality—our bodily dependence
on food, in turn, on the sustaining hand of the Creator who
designed the earth to bring forth food—daily reminds us of a
spiritual reality: our dependence on Christ.

—Rachel Marie Stone, *Eat With Joy*

I sat down with a drive-through salad in my lap. It was the best
decision I could make that day. A mold remediation team had
just torn apart our kitchen island, and within twenty-four hours,
everything shifted. Discovering mold was one of those life surprises
you don't plan for. Temporarily, it was going to be paper plates and
fast food until we could get a new kitchen island rebuilt in four weeks.

I poured a little dressing on top of my salad and thought about
the oils likely used in the dressing—*inflammatory*. Then I secured the
lid, shook the salad, and opened it to take my first bite. I wondered
how many weird things were sprayed on the conventional lettuce—
toxic. I got a bite of candied nut—*added sugar*. All of this passed
through my mind in a matter of seconds. A mental commentary
shaped by decades of nutrition research, health articles, and "clean
eating" rules.

I suspect most of us have a complicated relationship with food.
It takes up a lot of time! We have to eat, and that leads to so many

choices over and over again. We have to consider health, the ease of preparation, what tastes good, and what our kids will *actually* eat. A few years ago, I asked some friends what caused them the most mental overwhelm, and it was food—always the food.

On top of that, you layer in a million marketing messages trying to sell you a way to eat. It is so noisy and conflicting.

Understanding macronutrients, micronutrients, vitamins, minerals, calories, and how they affect our physiology can be fascinating and beneficial. I'll enthusiastically nerd out about those things with you.

However, here is the candid conversation we need to have: Marketing for weight loss diets, health books, and fitness programs relies on making you feel dissatisfied or fearful. These underlying emotions move people to action to sell whatever they are selling. Research shows that people are more likely to move away from what they don't want instead of towards what they do want. This principle is called loss aversion.

How does this relate to food? Many of us have been conditioned to see what's wrong with our food first and foremost, which has led to a distorted relationship with it. We have been focusing on the "problem" with our food.

The constant barrage of dietary advice and fear-based messaging can create a climate of anxiety and obsession. Even good and "healthy" practices, like eating enough protein, can morph into compulsive counting and control. Fixation becomes just as unhealthy as neglect.

Studies suggest that disordered eating often develops over years, reinforced by patterns of control and autonomy struggles rather than appearing suddenly.[27] None of us just wake up one day with an eating disorder; rather, we spend years seeing food and our bodies in a particular way, rehearsing independence and control over them.

---

27 Franziska V. Froreich et al., "Psychological Need Satisfaction, Control, and Disordered Eating," *British Journal of Clinical Psychology* 56, no. 1 (March 2017): 53–68, https://doi.org/10.1111/bjc.12120.

I sat there with my salad and intrusive thoughts, and a little tug in my spirit reminded me that God is sovereign even over my little salad. It seems obvious to say that. Of course, God is sovereign over it all, but I think we sometimes need the reminder—especially when we're trying to control every bite, every outcome, every unknown.

I haven't solved the mystery of free will and God's sovereignty. But I do know this: when we lean too hard in one direction, we lose the beauty of the tension. Scripture holds both. We are called to make wise choices (Ephesians 5:15–17), and we are also called to trust that God is working all things for His glory (Romans 8:28). We cannot know everything. And we were never meant to. I said grace and prayed that it would nourish my body, thanking God for every bite I was about to take.

As we enter the following chapters, we must remind ourselves of the fallout of pursuing human knowledge without God's wisdom. We can be nutrition experts, and we can still be unhealthy because our minds and our souls are undernourished. When we live with a Gospel vision for health, our bodies tell a different story. They aren't projects to perfect; they are places of worship. We practice this vision by living as Gospel-shaped bodies—bodies that reflect the pattern of dependence on Christ, connection through community, and integration of our mind, body, and soul.

Sometimes, we get so caught up in *what* to eat that we skip the bigger, eternal priorities—the truths shaped by *how* we eat. We know that eating healthy food is, well, healthy. It honors the body. It reflects stewardship. Healthy eating matters—but health isn't the same as holiness. If we jump to habits without addressing the heart, we end up with behavior change but not transformation. When we begin with belief, with truth, our habits become an overflow of something far more lasting.

Gratitude

If our vision for health is to first and foremost surrender it all to the work of the Lord, then gratitude is the most natural place to begin with food. **Gratitude for our food isn't just a ritual before we eat—it's a declaration of dependence.** It reorients us to the Creator who provides, reminding us that every bite is an act of grace and every meal is a chance to connect our whole selves with Him.

Despite loads of books, Instagram reels, and mom blogs telling you all the ways certain foods will destroy your health, food is not the villain. We've made it the enemy—something to fear, moralize, and master.

It's not just about what is good—it's about order. When we fixate on dietary rules and restrictions instead of fixing our eyes on Jesus, we disrupt the connections that make us whole and healthy, which always begins with Christ. When health becomes the pursuit of control rather than an act of faithfulness, we are no longer living in that order.

Gratitude offers a powerful antidote to this. It interrupts the narrative where food is a chore to manage or a problem to solve. When we shift our focus to gratitude, we counter the cultural norm. We reframe the moment. Food becomes more than calories or control. It becomes an opportunity to receive. It's a daily reminder that we are not the source. And by the very act of giving thanks, we name it for what it is: a gift.

We will repeatedly see that biblical principles are backed by science. Research consistently shows that gratitude positively impacts physical health, emotional stability, and even our relationships.[28] Simply, gratitude is healthy!

When we praise God for our food, we begin to rightly order our health. This doesn't mean that we don't consider *what* we eat, but it

---

28 Amy Morin, "7 Scientifically Proven Benefits of Gratitude," *Psychology To-day*, April 3, 2015, https://www.psychologytoday.com/us/blog/what-mental-ly-strong-people-dont-do/201504/7-scientifically-proven-benefits-of-gratitude.

does mean that when we forget to remember God's provision, we miss out on the eternal implications of our temporary condition.

Saying grace before a meal is not new or groundbreaking, and it's easy to go through the motions without truly grasping the profound meaning behind the simple act. Jesus, once again, sets the example for us when He teaches us to pray: "Give us today our daily bread" (Matthew 6:11). Daily bread is our sustenance, a symbol of God's faithfulness, and our recognition of His provision breaking into our ordinary days.

Gratitude is what transforms our routines into worship.

The scriptures weave the theme of bread all the way through the story—from manna in the wilderness to the broken loaf in the hands of Christ. There's a reason for that. As Norman Wirzba writes, "In the minds of many throughout time, without bread there simply is no life."[29]

Bread and life become synonymous—a picture of our physical and spiritual dependence. The first reminds us of our daily needs. Not a day goes by that we don't have to think about food. We recognize our dependence, surrender to God's sovereignty, and image Jesus as we humbly offer praise and gratitude. Every meal reminds us that Jesus is our daily bread—life through Him.

Shared Meals

Bread doesn't just nourish the individual; it brings people together. It reminds us that God's provision was always meant to be shared. The feeding of the 5,000 is the only miracle, aside from the resurrection, recorded in all four Gospels. We again see this theme of daily provision—Jesus teaches, and then he gives them fish and *bread*. Jesus provides both physical and spiritual nourishment.

But look closer. Jesus could have effortlessly snapped his fingers and produced a meal for the masses. He didn't do that. Instead, He entrusted His disciples with the task of distribution—communal

29 Norman Wirzba, *Food and Faith: A Theology of Eating* (New York: Cambridge University Press, 2011), 12, quoting H.E. Jacob, Six Thousand Years of Bread: Its Holy and Unholy History (New York: Lyons Press, 1944).

participation. When the disciples passed the bread and fish, they weren't just handing out food. They were stepping into the miracle. Each hand that reached out, each piece broken and given, became a thread in the fabric of connection. It wasn't logistics. It was relational.

Not only were they nourishing their bodies, but they were also engaging their physical selves in serving

> Then he took the five loaves and the two fish, and looking up to heaven, he blessed and broke them. He kept giving them to the disciples to set before the crowd.
>
> — Luke 9:16

others' physical needs—a demonstration of the interconnectedness between the Provider, the disciples, and the community. This is a beautiful picture of how Christ works through the church body to care for the human body.

As Justin Whitmel Earley writes in *The Common Rule*, "Food is meant to bind us to God, neighbor, and creation, but we live in a culture where our eating habits keep us apart and increase our isolation."[30] When we serve our neighbors or family a meal, we physically demonstrate a spiritual reality—we depend on one another.

Celebrating over a meal is a rehearsal of shared dependance and a tangible expression of connection.

Eating together meets two of our deepest needs: nourishment and belonging. In fact, research shows that gathering for family meals has an inverse relationship with the occurrence of eating disorders.[31] Can we take a moment to recognize how profound that is? Could togetherness be as important as the labels on your food? Could breaking bread, an act as old as time, be foundational to our health? Even our language reflects this truth. The word companion comes

30 Justin Whitmel Earley, *The Common Rule: Habits of Purpose for an Age of Distraction* (Downers Grove, IL: InterVarsity Press, 2019), 59.

31 Jess Haines et al., "Systematic Review of the Effects of Family Meal Frequency on Psychosocial Outcomes in Youth," *Canadian Family Physician* 61, no. 2 (February 2015): e96–e106, https://www.ncbi.nlm.nih.gov/pmc/articles/PMC4325878/.

from the Latin *com* ("with"), and *panis* ("bread")—a companion is one with whom you eat bread.[32]

Breaking bread has always been more than food—it is about relationship, dependence, and grace. Jamie Erickson reminds us in *Holy Hygge* that "All throughout the Gospels, we see Jesus building fellowship around a meal."[33] He began His ministry at a wedding banquet, and just before He went to the cross, He participated in the Last Supper with His disciples. Even in His resurrected, physical body, He broke bread (Luke 24:30-31).

Our relationship with food is shaped by the people we share it with.

I suspect you are the type of woman who will read this and immediately think of how you can serve your family, neighbors, and community well with food. That's beautiful! But I also want to remind you that this also means allowing yourself to be served a good meal.

When our kitchen was under mold remediation, friends offered to bring us meals, and I declined—worried that I was adding more to their already full plates. I later realized I was missing something. I wasn't just turning down a meal; I was turning down an opportunity for connection and sharing in each other's burdens and blessings.

It's natural for women, as moms and caretakers, to take on the role of giver. However, accepting a gift, especially a gift of a nourishing meal, is just as holy and good as serving one. It's an acknowledgment of our shared humanity, our mutual dependence, and our place within the body of Christ.

Wonder

One of my favorite ways to serve my family is to bake fresh bread. The aroma signals my boys to make their way to the kitchen, eagerly

---

32 Rachel Marie Stone, *Eat with Joy: Redeeming God's Gift of Food* (Downers Grove, IL: InterVarsity Press, 2013), 67

33 Jamie Erickson, *Holy Hygge: Creating a Place for People to Gather and the Gospel to Grow* (Chicago: Moody Publishers, 2022), 30.

anticipating those first warm slices generously coated in butter. Their joy in turn, fills me with purpose and fulfillment.

I hope someday, when they're older, the smell of fresh bread brings them back to those moments. To the kitchen. To remember that they were nourished, and they were loved.

When I bake bread, I'm reminded that feeding someone is never just about food. It's about presence, care, and provision. It's a small echo of how God meets us. Think about it: a handful of simple ingredients—flour, water, yeast—transformed by time, warmth, and a little human effort into a loaf of fragrant, nourishing bread. We call it ordinary. But it's not. It's holy work.

When Jesus calls Himself the Bread of Life, He isn't just offering sustenance; He is offering Himself—daily, abundantly, eternally. Our bodies need food to live. Our souls need Christ to live. And as we have also seen, Jesus feeds a multitude with bread. Christ is not so subtly calling us to understand that our physical realities point us to spiritual truths.

Every time we sit down to a meal, we are witnessing with our very eyes nothing short of a miracle. I don't know much about farming, but I have tried to grow a few vegetables before. The thing that I learned is that I can't make anything grow. It is this beautiful reliance on the sun, the ground, the seed, and the soil. It's God's goodness and grace that He has woven into His very creation. Whether we give Him glory or not, we are blessed through His creation.

We must eat to live, and by this very fact, we are nourished and strengthened not just by calories and nutrients but by the source of life that made our bodies and all of creation interdependent for life. Every meal, every loaf, every harvest is a small miracle pointing to the greatest miracle—the Word made flesh, broken and given for us. Every table whispers the story of the cross and the empty tomb.

Consider this: microscopic organisms breaking down what's old so something new can grow. Pollinators moving between plants, carrying life. Rain soaking the soil. Sunlight drawing seeds upward. Seasons shifting with unnoticed reliability. It's not random. It's a design woven with intention. A system built not just for survival, but for abundance. This is the work of a Creator who sees, who knows, who sustains. Let that settle.

If we truly grasped the wonder of it all, every meal would be a celebration of praise.

Preparing and eating a meal can be reframed from a chore and overwhelming choices to a chance at gratitude, togetherness, and wonder multiple times a day. We can rewrite the anxious thoughts telling us that our food is another problem to control. We can begin to see our food as a gift, transforming our daily meals into moments of connection, gratitude, and awe. Deeply meaningful liturgies such as saying grace and breaking bread together reorient our affections, grounding us in practices that nourish our bodies, hearts, and minds through connection.

Whether it's a drive-through salad providing quick nourishment amid chaos or a table full of warm bread, every meal is a reminder to taste and see that the Lord is good (Psalm 34:8).

The Heart of It

Christ Connection: When food becomes a source of fear or control, the Gospel reminds us to begin with gratitude—seeing each meal as provision from the One who calls Himself the Bread of Life.

Community Connection: Shared meals are more than nutrition—they are communion, a sacred act of giving and receiving that binds us to one another and reveals the heart of God.

Whole Body Connection: We don't just eat to live—we eat to remember, to rejoice, to reflect our dependence on God in body and soul, allowing every meal to be both sustenance and worship.

7

Movement

How do we align exercise with the Gospel vision of health?

"Each morning is an opportunity to praise God as the giver of life. Does your life shout 'God is my creator! I am the clay, the work of his hand!' (Isa. 64:8)? Are you overwhelmed by the gift of your beating heart, the breath in your lungs, the blood pumping through your veins, and your intricate immune system? They are all a part of his glorious design. Isn't life itself an invitation to worship him for how wonderfully he made you?"

—Lindsey Carlson, *Identity Theft* (2019), 117.

In November 2012, I ran the Turkey Trot with my husband. Running had been a part of my life for years—cross-country in high school, half marathons in adulthood, and plenty of Turkey Trots in between.

A couple of miles into the race, I stopped to walk. I felt heavy, and my body felt *different*. My husband was perplexed, and frankly, I was confused and frustrated with my body. I had always been able to push—one foot in front of the other.

I discovered in junior high that running was one way to exercise my dissatisfaction with my body. I could punish it by pushing, going farther and faster. I thought I loved running because it gave me a feeling of control and an outlet for my anger and frustration. If I didn't like how I looked that day. Run. If I ate a little too much. Run. If there was something outside my control that happened that day. Run.

I genuinely believed this was a "healthy" outlet. After all, running is healthy, right? Our culture tends to judge the behavior, not the motive. If the activity looks good on the outside, we rarely question what's driving it. When I couldn't control other things, I could be the boss of my body. It's more socially acceptable to over-exercise than to turn to substances to numb, but let me be clear—I was still numbing through a false sense of control.

I've been asked more times than I can count: What's the best kind of exercise? But that's never been the right question. The better question is: how are you doing the exercise, and why? The same is true of our spiritual posture towards movement. Exercise is never neutral. It's either something that aligns our hearts with Christ, or it's something that fuels false narratives we are trying to unlearn.

This verse in Colossians 3:23 reframes how we view our physical habits as spiritual practices: "Whatever you do, do it from the heart, as something done for the Lord and not for people." And once we see it, we stop asking *what* kind of exercise is best and start asking *how* we're doing it and *why* it matters.

By the grace of God, I listened to my body. I released control and walked. A week later, I took a pregnancy test and found out I was pregnant with my first son. That Thanksgiving Day would be my last time running for a decade.

Movement is part of a healthy body and life. That is undeniable. We want more energy, improved focus and cognition, and lower stress levels. Exercise can significantly improve all these things. The research is vast and compelling. According to a University of Georgia study, low-intensity exercise can lower symptoms of fatigue and increase energy levels by 20%.[34]

Yet we spend billions every year trying to buy what our bodies were designed to create.

---

34 Sam Fahmy, "Low-Intensity Exercise Reduces Fatigue Symptoms by 65 Percent, Study Finds," *UGA Today*, February 28, 2008, https://news.uga.edu/low-intensity-exercise-reduces-fatigue-symptoms-by-65-percent-study-finds/.

In 2023, the global energy drink market reached nearly $193 billion,[35] and the energy supplement market is projected to grow to $152.5 billion by 2031.[36]

And in 2023, Americans spent 301 million PER DAY on coffee and related goods.[37] And so we're clear, I'm not coming for your coffee. I'd lose all credibility if I pretended I didn't have a standing date with my morning cold brew.

Health, once the fruit of faithfulness and embodied care, has become a consumer activity. We don't live it; we purchase pieces of it.

However, moving our bodies is free. Movement benefits our physical, emotional, and mental health. But if we don't pause to evaluate our posture toward it, we unknowingly use exercise as a means of striving rather than a practice of stewardship.

I stopped running—not because running is bad, but because I needed to redeem my relationship with it.

Stewardship

We must consider our hearts before we lace up our running shoes, throw on our workout clothes, or pick up a dumbbell. For me, exercise was a way to feel in control. Maybe for others it's something to check off a list—just another task. For some, it becomes an idol—where worth seems to hang on a number, a routine, or a result. Either way, we are called to something more. We are committed to living differently, fully embracing what it means to inhabit our bodies purposefully.

Dreading or idolizing your workouts will not lead to wholeness— physically or spiritually. It deepens the divide between body and soul. The *just do it* mentality comes from a secular mindset prioritizing

35 Statista, "Energy Drinks – Worldwide," *Statista Research Department*, 2023, https://www.statista.com/topics/10313/energy-drinks-worldwide/.

36 Allied Market Research, "Energy Supplement Market," August 2022, https://www.alliedmarketresearch.com/energy-supplement-market-A16879.

37 Nick Brown, "Report: Daily U.S. Coffee Consumption Hits 20-Year High," *Daily Coffee News*, April 12, 2024, https://dailycoffeenews.com/2024/04/12/report-daily-us-coffee-consumption-hits-20-year-high/.

control and performance over connection. But as we've already established, a Gospel-shaped body is one of integration, not separation.

> If we live by the Spirit, let us also keep in step with the Spirit.
> —Galatians 5:25

Self-control is a fruit of the Spirit, not a badge of performance. It means we sometimes move even when we don't feel like it because it is good. Our culture praises self-discipline in exercise as a personal achievement. **But in Christ, discipline is always rooted in devotion.** Some days, moving your body in faithfulness is an act of worship, even when it costs you comfort. And that difference—between striving and stewardship—makes all the difference.

What if exercise wasn't just about discipline, but also about delight?

When I watch my kids, I see a different kind of movement. They don't run, play, swim, or climb trees because they are self-disciplined. They move for the joy of it. It's instinctive because they were made for it.

My boys and I watched a documentary called *Riot and the Dance*, and one scene captured a humpback whale breaching. Watching an animal of that size launch itself out of the water was breathtaking. Why do they do it? Scientists have many theories, but one is simple: for the joy of it. Because they *can*. Sometimes, we move in faith, trusting that joy often follows obedience. Other times, we move for the joy of it—simply because we can.

What brings you joy? If you love music, put on a playlist and dance—or run to the beat. Competitive? Sign up for a race or set a new personal best. Take your workout outside and move under the open sky if you love the outdoors. None of these things in themselves is more holy than the other. What makes your workout holy is your heart's posture towards it.

When movement becomes an expression of worship, we glorify God and image Christ to the world.

I can't tell you whether Pilates is better than barre or weightlifting is better than running for you right now in your season. But I can tell you this: If your movement does not bring you into deeper alignment with your vision for health and holiness, it's time to rethink it. Our bodies were created to move—but even more, they were created to reflect Christ in how we live, serve, and move through the world.

When we embrace movement as worship, we are not just stewarding strength or endurance. We are embodying the fruit of the Spirit—imaging Christ in every step, every stretch, every act of faithfulness, whether it flows from joy or is formed through discipline.

It's not just about what your body can do, it's about Who your body reflects in the process.

Shared Life

A few years ago, my husband and I, inspired by the 75-hard trend, decided to take a daily walk together outside. It has turned into a time for us to catch up, get some sunshine, pray, share projects we are working on with each other, and move our bodies. It became less about the steps we logged and more about our conversations. Movement has the power to create these kinds of shared memories because it draws us to the present moment.

While preparing for this chapter, I came across a familiar idea in a wellness book: the belief that *your fitness journey is for you alone.* At first, it didn't even register as unusual. After all, this messaging is everywhere. But when I paused to consider it, I realized how deeply it reflects how our culture views health. It's a common theme in fitness and wellness: *your body, your goals, your journey.* While it fuels an industry built on personal transformation, it misses something essential. Health isn't just personal; it's communal. Because *we* are communal.

Movement is good for the body. But it's even better when it's together. Research shows that exercising in a group is even more effective in reducing stress than working out alone.[38] It also makes movement more sustainable over the long run.[39] But beyond statistics, we know this intuitively. When movement is woven into our relationships, it becomes more than just a habit. It becomes a place where joy is cultivated and connection is strengthened.

Movement is a means of presence—with God, with others, and with our bodies.

Whether you give God the glory or not, exercise benefits the body because it is a part of God's grace and goodness in His design. But if our motivation is weight loss, looking more toned, or fitting into a particular pair of jeans, we're chasing something temporary. There's nothing wrong with temporary goals, but they will never give us the fullness of life we long for. Exercise takes on eternal significance when it strengthens us to hold our children, care for the sick, and create lasting memories through shared movement.

Years from now, we won't remember the number on the scale. We'll remember the walks. The bike rides. The hikes. The races. The hands we held and the memories we made because we chose to move together. We won't remember what we did as much as who we did it with.

Strength

At first glance, exercise may seem the least spiritual of all the topics in this book. After all, we do it to strengthen our bodies—muscles, bones, immune systems, hearts, and minds. But as followers of Christ, we know this: everything we do in our bodies matters. Every act has spiritual significance. Because everything is sacred.

38 Dayna M. Yorks, Christopher A. Frothingham, and Mark D. Schuenke, "Effects of Group Fitness Classes on Stress and Quality of Life of Medical Students," *Journal of the American Osteopathic Association* 117, no. 11 (November 2017): e17–e25, https://doi.org/10.7556/jaoa.2017.140.

39 P.A. Estabrooks, "Sustaining Exercise Participation Through Group Cohesion," *Exercise and Sport Sciences Reviews* 28, no. 2 (April 2000): 63–67, https://pubmed.ncbi.nlm.nih.gov/10902087/.

Still, we've absorbed a cultural lens that often isolates exercise from the rest of life. Dr. Casey Means puts words to this disconnect.

"I believe the answer lies in the fundamental concept of 'exercise.' We have characterized exercise as an isolated bout of activity—separate from the rest of our daily life—an item on the to-do list. Our metabolic processes function best when movement is a regular, consistent part of our lives, not a task to be performed in an hour or two."[40]

She points to a truth woven into our humanity. Movement is an essential. Just as we are made for dependence, community, integration, and receiving nourishment outside of ourselves, we are also made for motion.

Exercise is as good for the soul as it is for the body—because it draws us back into how we were meant to live.

That might look like walking with your spouse while praying over your life and children.

Or maybe it's challenging yourself to lift heavier weights with friends cheering you on so you can carry your babies with strength.

It might mean joining a fitness class and forming new friendships.

Or doing gentle stretches on your living room floor while your newborn naps, praising God for the body that brought life into the world.

Maybe, just maybe, it's lacing up your running shoes for the first time in ten years—not to prove something, but to run with your pre-teen boys. For the memories. The laughter. And yes, even the struggle. Because it's the connection that makes it holy.

How we move our bodies, with joy, with others, and with regularity matters, but we must always keep the why in clear focus. We are no longer exercising to chase after a distorted image of cultural beauty. The issue isn't movement itself; it's the motivation beneath it. If our workouts are driven by fear, dissatisfaction, or the desire to control our bodies, they can expose an idol—whether that's

---

40 Casey Means, MD, and Calley Means, *Good Energy: The Surprising Connection Between Metabolism and Limitless Health* (New York: Avery Publishing Group, 2024), 213.

beauty, approval, or self-sufficiency. But when we move as an act of stewardship, honoring the body God has given us, exercise becomes an act of worship rather than a pursuit of perfection.

We move our bodies as a practice to continue to lay down our ease of life to build strength and resilience. We move because it is a part of who we are. Because when we do it with a heart posture of wanting to steward our lives and bodies well, we worship Christ for the gift of life He has given us. And as we continue to practice building bodily resilience, it helps us to learn to develop our mental, spiritual, and emotional resilience.

The Heart of It

Christ Connection: When our discipline is rooted in devotion, movement becomes more than exercise; it becomes worship, done from the heart, for the Lord.

Community Connection: Movement becomes holy when it creates shared presence, strengthens relationships, and turns everyday moments into eternal ones.

Whole Body Connection: Exercise is not just a physical act—it is a spiritual formation in motion, reinforcing joy, building resilience, and embodying the truth that everything we do in our bodies matters to God.

8

Resilience

How do we align stress management
with the Gospel vision of health?

Resilience is the ability to be content, to accept what is, and to have
the courage to surrender to Christ anything that comes our way.

—Rebekah Lyons, *Building a Resilient Life*

Twenty years ago, I was sitting in a college class on *Stress Management* when I first heard a stat that stopped me in my track:

60–80% of all doctors' visits are stress-related.

The lecture continued, explaining that stress is a contributing factor in nearly every ailment we experience. At that moment, I thought I had discovered the answer.

My 20-something brain interpreted that as a clear directive: *Just don't be stressed!* Problem solved, right? I believed the answers were out there in the data, the research, or in someone else's expertise. Some key that would explain how to live in this body and not feel frustrated by what it couldn't do or scared of losing what it could do.

At that moment, it felt like I'd cracked the code to staying healthy. Avoid stress, and you'll be fine. Simple.

It *is* simple. But simple doesn't mean easy. The older I get, the more I realize how the solution "don't be stressed" can become its own source of pressure.

The problem with stats like the one I shared above (and we see loads of cherry-picked stats like this, especially on social media) is that they stress us out. Why? Because single data points are designed to motivate us into action—but without context, they distort the bigger picture. We end up obsessing over narrow solutions while missing the deeper story. Instead of clarity, they leave us carrying the heavy burden of trying to control the impossible.

The reality is we will encounter stress regularly. It shows up in the daily moments: breaking up sibling fights, facing tight deadlines, sitting in traffic (when we needed to be somewhere fifteen minutes ago), or getting news that upends our plans. And sometimes, we face adversities marked by pain, grief, and fear.

If we believe our goal is to avoid stress, adversity, and all the emotions that come with it, then we are going to be constantly on the run. If you have read a health book on stress, there is almost always a description of our bodies in fight-or-flight mode where a bear or a tiger is chasing us. This illustration is used to help us understand what happens to our bodies under stress, and it is also a demonstration that we aren't supposed to always be on the run. The irony is that we have all been running from stress itself. We have been running scared and haven't been able to get a break from it.

Wild animals aren't chasing us, but we have been living as if they are—constantly running from stress as if escape is the answer. But what if we stopped running? What if instead we stood firm in faith?

Most of the advice we hear today treats stress like an enemy to be avoided at all costs. "Eliminate stress." "Live a stress-free life." "Cut out anything that doesn't serve you." These are the messages we see over and over again. The problem? A life without stress doesn't exist. More importantly, Scripture never frames stress as something to run from, and we don't ever see Jesus telling His disciples to avoid stress—nor do we see Him modeling that.

While Jesus never warned us against stress itself, He did have something to say about worry in Matthew 6:25. "Therefore, I tell you, don't **worry** about your life, what you will eat or what you will drink, or about your body, what you will wear. Isn't life more than food and the body more than clothing?"

In Greek, the word for worry, also sometimes translated as anxiety, is *merimnaō*. This word is related to the word *merizō*, which means to divide, to separate into parts, cut into pieces, to disunite.[41]

Right before this statement, Jesus talked about being unable to serve two masters. It's about resisting the pull to split ourselves between competing priorities.

Do you see it? **The problem isn't the stress. The problem is the divided heart and mind.**

That's why it's important to distinguish between stress and anxiety. Stress is a natural, and even sometimes necessary, response to challenge. Anxiety is defined as a persistent, internal fear that isn't always tied to a specific cause. Both deserve attention, but this chapter is about the daily stresses we all carry—and how to live through them in a way that keeps us whole.

We're not trying to escape stress. We're learning how to move through it with resilience. And that's something we can practice.

Stress can be a good thing in many cases. Stress leads to growth. As we have already discussed, exercise is stress on the body, which builds resilience in the body. Likewise, sickness is a stress that can build resilience in the immune system. When we learn something new, we stress the brain, stimulating neuroplasticity for it to form new pathways.

But stress is not only physical. It is emotional and spiritual, too. Our beliefs about it shape our biology just as much as our behaviors. Perhaps this is why James begins his writings to us with: "Consider it a great joy, my brothers and sisters, whenever you experience trials because you know the testing of your faith produces endurance" (James 1:2). The goal is to face stress and adversity in a way that builds us, not breaks us.

Throughout His ministry, Jesus met both physical and spiritual needs, but not always in the same order. When He healed the paralytic (Matthew 9:2-7), He first said, "Your sins are forgiven," addressing the man's spiritual need before restoring his body. But when He fed

---

41 *Bible Hub*, HELPS Word-Studies, s.v. "Merimnaó (Strong's 3309)," https://bible-hub.com/greek/3309.htm

the 5,000 (John 6:1-35), He provided physical sustenance first, then pointed them to Himself as the Bread of Life.

Likewise, in our own lives, there are times when tending to the body first—through rest, nourishment, or movement—creates space for the quiet our minds and souls need. Other times, beginning with Scripture and prayer reorders our affections and changes how we approach everything else. Either way, true peace is only found in connection to Christ.

I spent years focused on mitigating stress through the body— better sleep, better nutrition, better movement. These things matter. But during a semester-long project in my stress management class, I realized what was missing. We were assigned to pick a behavior to change, research it, create a plan, and track it. I chose to quit coffee—which is hilarious now, sitting here in a coffee shop, sipping cold brew as I share this story.

Not only did I fail to quit coffee by the end of the semester; I didn't even quit temporarily. The class focused on changing behavior, but it never addressed belief.

And that's the missing piece for so many of us. Before we launch into a to-do list of stress management strategies, we must begin by redefining our relationship to stress.

Connection over Consumption

When stress hits, most of us instinctively reach for something to comfort us, make us feel better, and help us find relief. Sometimes we confuse consumption with connection. In times of stress, we tend to consume social media, Netflix, food, alcohol, or shopping— almost all of these fall into the numbing category. When we consume instead of connect, we move away from being embodied. It is an escape. There is temporary relief as we suspend reality, but when we return to our routines, we haven't done anything to move ourselves forward. Over time, we become stuck in our stress, and we inhibit our resilience.

In a compilation of essays on resilience by the *Harvard Business Review*, one author identified three themes that consistently appeared in people and organizations able to recover from adversity.[42] The first was the ability to see and accept reality for what it truly is. When we turn to escapism or numbing to cope, we bypass this critical starting point. We trade the chance to grow for the illusion of relief. True resilience can only be built by living in what's real.

Prayer brings us fully into the present *and* Christ's presence. When we acknowledge the true state of our struggles and bring them to God, something deeper happens. Prayer demands connection.

Prayer pulls us into reality rather than away from it. It reminds us of our dependence, reorders our affections, and engages our whole selves. We use our minds to reflect, our mouths to speak, and our bodies to kneel or lift our hands. It's not just spiritual—it's physical. It requires all of us.

We can bring ourselves before the Lord through Christ at any moment. Yet we often settle for spinning in our thoughts—replaying what we can't control, obsessing over what we fear. And when those thoughts become too much to bear, we check out. We disconnect. We numb. We avoid seeing reality for what it truly is because escape feels like the only relief we can access.

We forget the sacred practices that connect us—not just to calm, but to Christ. Not just to ourselves, but to our Creator: the Prince of Peace (Isaiah 9:6), the Bread of Life (John 6:35), Emmanuel (Matthew 1:23), the Light of the World (John 8:12), the Good Shepherd (John 10:11), the Rock (1 Corinthians 10:4). These names are not just poetic. They are deeply personal. Each one speaks to how Jesus meets us in our stress and offers something far better than relief: He offers Himself.

Some of us, on the other hand, have what look like productive coping mechanisms. When stress hits, we reach for another supplement, a new app, a better planner, or the latest meal-prep service. We believe the marketing. *This next thing* will finally make

---

42 Diane L. Coutu, "How Resilience Works," *Harvard Business Review* 80, no. 5 (May 2002): 46–50, 52, 55, https://hbr.org/2002/05/how-resilience-works.

everything feel manageable. But more often than not, we already have what we need. We have access to the One who holds all things together (Colossians 1:17).

Stress management techniques like breath-work, guided reflections, and journaling bring us into the present moment by engaging both the body and the mind. They work because they move us toward connection and support us in meaningful ways.

But even the best of them can only take us so far. They fall short of the kind of transformation that produces lasting peace. They connect us to ourselves—but not to the One who gives peace that endures. That kind of peace can only come from the mind of Christ, and it can only be accessed through connection with Him.

> **But seek first the kingdom of God and his righteousness, and all these things will be provided for you.**
>
> **— Matthew 6:33**

This is why Jesus doesn't say, "Seek better tools." He says, "Seek the kingdom of God." Because tools can support, but they're not the source.

Together

Stress was never meant to be carried solo—but many of us try. The church body wasn't just a clever metaphor when Paul called the wholeness of professing followers of Christ—*the body*. It is a profound reality. As discussed, we represent the physical presence of Christ in this world, but this presence was always meant to be a group project.

We often imagine the church body through the lens of Sunday morning—worship, sermons, and shared space. But the body of Christ was never intended to be confined to a service. It was meant to show up on our Mondays, our text threads, on our meal trains, and in our moments of unraveling. It's not just how we gather. It's how we live.

Research has shown that support from others doesn't just help us emotionally; it changes how we perceive difficulty. In one study, participants estimated a hill to be less steep when they stood with a close friend. Even imagining someone supportive made the hill feel less daunting than picturing someone neutral or unkind. The presence of support made the path ahead feel more manageable.[43]

Isn't that exactly what God intended the body of Christ to be? **When we walk together, the climb doesn't disappear, but it no longer feels impossible.**

We learn who we are by walking alongside others. We also find the strength of our resilience is directly tied to the strength of our relationships. Many of us struggle with this. We try to carry everything ourselves—our responsibilities, our stress, our burdens—as if we are meant to be the whole body rather than just a part of it. And wholeness requires connection. Paul describes the church as a body with many members, each with different gifts and roles (1 Corinthians 12:12-27). When we attempt to do everything on our own, we step outside of what it looks like imaging Christ, which inhibits our ability to learn, grow, and recover from stress.

The metaphor of the church body mirrors the way God designed the human body itself. When we look at how cells function, we see why no part of the body was meant to operate alone. Every cell has a job—carrying oxygen, fighting infection, repairing tissue. Health happens when each cell contributes, doing what it was made to do.

But when a cell begins to operate independently, ignoring the needs of the body, disorder follows. Cancer forms when cells multiply without restraint, consuming instead of contributing—harming the very body that gives them life. The body can't thrive when one part tries to do it all, and it breaks down when its parts begin to work against each other.[44]

---

43 Simone Schnall et al., "Social Support and the Perception of Geographical Slant," *Journal of Experimental Social Psychology* 44, no. 5 (September 2008): 1246–1255, https://doi.org/10.1016/j.jesp.2008.04.011.

44 Stephen Ko, *Faith Embodied* (Grand Rapids, MI: Zondervan, 2025), 5.

This is more than an interesting insight. It reveals something deeper: unity and interdependence are how God works—and how He formed us to live. When we remember we are only *part* of the body, we can embrace both our limitations and our need for others.

Resilience isn't just about surviving stress. It's about being transformed through it—together. God uses struggle to strengthen us and deepen our dependence on Him and our connection to each other. That might look like bearing burdens through prayer, sharing a meal, or just sitting in silence with someone in pain. Sometimes it's as simple as showing up—and staying.

We don't just endure stress; we are formed by it.

Meaning

We don't usually associate stress with purpose. Most of us just want relief from it. But what if stress isn't something to avoid or push through, but something God can use to reshape us?

What if we returned to what James tells us, and began to see our stress and adversity—*as joy?* Not because hardship is easy or enjoyable, but because it has a purpose.

Ruth Chou Simons explains this beautifully in *Now and Not Yet*: "When we feel angst, instability, or restlessness, our brains are activated to learn something it would otherwise ignore." In other words, difficulty isn't just something to *survive*. It's a catalyst for growth. Neuroscience confirms this: studies on neuroplasticity show that it's challenge, not comfort, that rewires the brain and builds resilience. As Simons notes, stability can actually shut down the learning process.[45]

Reframing stress has benefits. Instead of avoiding it, we can see it as God's way of refining us. Rather than something to suppress or escape, stress, when anchored in truth, becomes a tool for transformation.

---

45 Ruth Chou Simons, *Now and Not Yet: Pressing in When You're Waiting, Wanting, and Restless for More* (Nashville: Thomas Nelson, 2024), 91.

Earlier, we looked at the *Harvard Business Review* article outlining three common patterns in resilient people. We've already explored the first—accepting reality. The second is just as crucial: resilient people are able to find meaning in their adversity.

The beauty of our faith is that we know the end of the story. The Christian story has the ultimate happy ending. We'll explore that ending later, but for now, we can rest in this: whatever trials we face, God will ultimately use them for good. The Christian life is resilient by its very nature when we return to the truth of what we believe, and when we remember who we are.

Finding meaning in our struggle is not a call to endure chaos at all costs. There's wisdom in evaluating our relationships, responsibilities, and rhythms and recognizing unhealthy trends in our lives. Some things need to be released. However, that wisdom must be held in tension with the willingness to embrace the struggles and stresses that are a natural part of life.

Christ often holds together what we'd rather separate—mercy and justice, divinity and humanity, death and life. Following Him means learning to live inside those tensions too. Wisdom doesn't always mean escape. Sometimes, it means staying—and being shaped.

The final theme in the HBR essay was this: resilient people know how to adapt. They work with what they have, adjust to reality, and turn obstacles into opportunities. Isn't that exactly what faith invites us to do? While the world tells us to consume, control, or avoid, faith calls us to trust, wait, and walk forward even when the path is unclear.

Resilience isn't just about survival. Despite all the stories about our ancestors running from bears and tigers, it's about seeing what's in our hands, however small or insufficient, and trusting that God can use it. It's taking the next step—not because we have everything we think we need, but because we believe He is enough.

Stress is inevitable. Jesus never told us to avoid it. He warned against being divided by it.

The world tells us to manage stress by numbing or controlling it, but resilience isn't about escaping stress; it's about facing it in a way that builds our faith and connections.

Most stress management strategies focus on one part of the equation—caring for our physical health or addressing our mental health. Some of these tools are helpful and even necessary. Others offer only temporary relief. But all of them fall short when they're disconnected from the lasting sources of peace we were created for.

The biblical model is holistic. Stress isn't something to manage in isolation but something to bring into alignment. It's meant to connect us more fully to God's strength, our relationships, and our spiritual formation. That includes honoring how we were created to function physically. Our bodies need rest, movement, nourishment, sunshine, water, and presence. When we neglect those basic needs, our ability to respond to stress, emotionally and spiritually, begins to break down.

We build resilience by aligning with God's design: staying connected to Christ, rooted in community, and attuned to the rhythms our bodies were made to follow.

The Heart of It

Christ Connection: Jesus doesn't offer escape—He offers Himself. In prayer, we move from consuming to connection. Peace doesn't come from tools or strategies. It comes from the One who is peace.

Community Connection: Just like the human body, the church body is healthier when each part shows up. Resilience isn't self-reliance—it's shared strength.

Whole Body Connection: Finding meaning in our stress reshapes us. When our beliefs align with how we care for our bodies, stress becomes more than something to manage—it becomes a place where growth takes root.

9

Rest

How do we align rest with the Gospel vision of health?

But at the heart of worship is rest—a stopping from all work, all worry, all scheming, all fleeing—to stand amazed and thankful before God and His work. There can be no real worship without true rest.

—Mark Buchanan, *The Rest of God*

I was nineteen, hunched over a desk in the back office of a 24-Hour Fitness, paper bag in hand, trying to catch my breath. Payroll had to be sent, but the operations manager, who usually handled it, was out for plastic surgery. A night-shift employee didn't show up, so I manned the gym by myself through the night.

After being up for over 24 hours, running on sheer willpower, the carrier left without the payroll sheets. My mind shut down. My heart raced. I couldn't breathe. I panicked. *Every employee was depending on me.*

I don't remember how it was resolved. I do remember the feeling when I realized my usual "I've got this" wasn't enough. My body had hit its limit, whether I admitted it or not.

At first, it might sound ironic. A gym is where people relieve stress, get stronger, and become the healthiest version of themselves. But for me? It became the place where my body finally said *enough*.

I brought the same mindset and naivety into the next job. This time, I wasn't inside the gym. I was on the road, driving home after a shift that went after hours in the lead-up to a grand opening at

Lifetime Fitness. My vision blurred. My chest tightened. I couldn't get enough air. I pulled over to the side of the road alone, gasping.

In hindsight, the pattern is painfully obvious. Both times, I was managing departments at large fitness chains that were open 24/7. I was working at places that never closed. They never stopped operating, and neither did I. Burnout wasn't a buzzword yet, but I was living it.

Burnout isn't just a personal struggle; it's a pervasive issue, particularly among women. Recent research indicates that women are disproportionately affected by chronic stress and burnout, often due to the compounded pressures of professional duties and societal roles.[46]

I was surrounded by a culture obsessed with pushing harder, working longer, and being the boss of your body—mind over matter. But there I was, physically shutting down. My body was rejecting everything I was telling it to do. Because here's the truth: the body isn't made to run 24 hours. Even my youth wasn't enough to overcome my humanity. My body needed rest.

The word *restoration* comes from the Latin root *restaurare*—to repair, rebuild, or renew. And restoration doesn't happen without rest.

Burnout isn't just my story. It's a pattern we've absorbed from a culture that celebrates exhaustion and calls it ambition. But underneath the overwork is a belief—a heart posture—that needs to be realigned.

The Heart of Rest

Everything we've talked about—health, movement, nourishment, resilience—it all begins and ends here: rest in Christ.

Rest is something we long for. We talk about needing it, plan for it, even pray for it. But it's still hard to find. Why? Because we think

---

46 Tait Shanafelt et al., "Changes in Burnout and Satisfaction With Work-Life Integration in Physicians and the General US Working Population Between 2011 and 2021," *JAMA Network Open* 5, no. 11 (November 2022): e2239346. https://doi.org/10.1001/jamanetworkopen.2022.39346.

rest is something we *do*. Or more specifically, something we *don't* do. **But the heart of rest isn't about activity. It's about belief.**

When Jesus uttered the words, "It is finished," (John 19:30), it was the climax of every one of our stories. It was the moment we saw how every conflict would be resolved, and Who would resolve it.

We often think of His death and resurrection in terms of eternity, salvation, and heaven. But His work on the cross doesn't just secure our future; it reshapes our present. It seeps into every part of our lives as we walk out our faith, including how we live, how we work, and how we rest.

"Come to me, all of you who are weary and burdened, and I will give you rest." (Matthew 11:28)

It's a well-known verse. We've heard it often enough to recite it, yet it hasn't always reached our hearts or settled into our bodies. Because we often miss what it's really saying: We can't come to Jesus *and* continue toiling away. You can't take on His rest *and* still carry your own weight.

Remember the wildflowers? Jesus has been telling us from the beginning that His kingdom doesn't operate like the world does. We don't work *for* rest; our work now flows *from* rest.

We don't have to be an outcome focused people, because we already know the outcome. We don't carry the weight because He carried the weight. This is both a past tense and a present tense situation. Our past is secured, and our present sustained.

We are instead a faithful people. Our work is now restful work because Jesus essentially said to us: *Come to me. Learn from me. Follow me.* (Matthew 4:19, John 10:27, John 8:12)

> My sheep hear my voice, I know them, and they follow me.
> —John 10:27

That means we don't have to obsess over outcomes. We don't have to fear getting it wrong or missing the plan. Our steps are ordered. Our path is lit. We don't rest because we've figured everything out.

We rest because Jesus went before us. A heart posture of rest is by no means passive or effortless; rather, it is an active expression of faith.

We can rest our bodies. We can quiet our minds. But until your heart is at rest in the finished work of Christ, you will never know the full restorative power of rest on this side of redemption.

The Culture of Rest

Rest is a shared rhythm. And it's within the community that we often learn how to rest, or more often than not, how not to rest. Rest is personal, but everything we do and don't do touches the lives of those around us. Our communities both shape our identity, and what we do also shapes our communities.

There are so many work cultures where the unspoken rule is to push harder, always. Give more than you have. Give 110%. Church communities, where rest should be the foundation, can sometimes esteem overextending oneself as a mark of spirituality. Similarly, in motherhood, there's often an unspoken expectation to do it all, misconstruing self-sacrifice as a virtue while neglecting personal well-being. We have a great calling within our communities; therefore, we twist this idea to mean that we should say yes to everything. We misunderstand what it means to be a living sacrifice. We convince ourselves that burnout is a mark of a well-lived life.

This mindset is cultural, not biblical. The secular ethos of "go big or go home" or "leave it all on the table" stems from a performance-based mentality where individuals are in the driver's seat, attempting to control outcomes through sheer effort. While striving for excellence is commendable, defining excellence through a biblical lens is crucial. True excellence aligns with the fruits of the Spirit—love, joy, peace, patience, kindness, goodness, faithfulness, gentleness, and self-control (Galatians 5:22). Work is an overflow from a heart of rest.

Running yourself into the ground doesn't serve anyone. In a way, we are saying with our actions that we are the ones that hold it all together. The research shows otherwise: a study published in the *Scandinavian Journal of Work, Environment & Health* found that productivity declines beyond a certain number of work hours. This demonstrates that overwork doesn't equal effectiveness.[47] Whereas, when we allow our heart posture of rest to ground the culture of our communities, we defiantly say, we trust the Lord fully. We trust in the work of Christ so much that we are going to honor His ways, His example, and His timing. We will rest whether we know it will all come together or not.

If you want to love your communities well, rest. Say no to the things that will overextend you. Demonstrate with your actions that you are a part of the body of Christ, not the whole body. Get comfortable living within your limits, and visibly walk out your trust in Jesus to fill the gaps. Let your kids see you model this, shift your church culture to align with the biblical mindset of dependence, and work His way, allowing space for God to restore your mind, your body, and your soul. Amen?

The Practice of Rest

We've explored how rest shapes our hearts and communities, but how do we actively learn to rest? We practice. We rest with our bodies so our hearts remember the truth. Although the Sabbath was an Old Testament law, it remains embedded in our design.

Sleep is one of the clearest reflections of this truth. It's a daily act of surrender, where our bodies heal and restore without our effort. In the same way, Sabbath rest reorients our souls through stillness. Both are rhythms that remind us: restoration begins with release, not effort. It's something God does in us.

"Numerous studies link the chronic lack of sleep (defined as less than six hours per night) with genetic damage, cardiovascular disease (such as hypertension and strokes), cancer, diabetes, infections, and inflammatory disorders such as rheumatoid arthritis. Chronic sleep

47 Kuroda S, Yamamoto I. "Does overwork decrease productivity? Evidence from panel data on Japanese workers." *Scand J Work Environ Health*. 2023;49(2):138–146. https://doi.org/10.5271/sjweh.4066

deprivation is also associated with infertility and even obesity, with sleep loss triggering increased hunger and a desire for high-calorie foods. Far from sleep being a waste of time, it plays an essential role in the daily restoration of damaged body components and a major role in prevention of disease."[48]

In other words, rest is a requirement to honor how we were made. It's both biological and theological. It is also modeled by Christ. We see Him sleeping in the middle of literal storms (Mark 4:37–39). That is a vivid picture of the rest He calls us to.

Biblical rest isn't just about stopping everything. It's about deliberately returning our focus to the One who sustains us. It's choosing to shut down at night, not because everything is finished, but because it never will be—and still, His provision is enough. It's saying no, even to good things, because faithfulness isn't about doing everything; it's about doing what He's called you to do.

Rest is a discipline—so we practice.

Many of us have become adept at incorporating good habits into our routines. Habits are actions we perform automatically, becoming part of our subconscious routines. For instance, going to bed at the same time each night, attending church every Sunday, or setting an alarm for a morning quiet time can evolve into habits.

However, Sabbath rest is a practice. And practices take presence—purposeful reflection, attention, and conscious *effort*. They aren't automatic. This distinction may explain why, despite setting ourselves up for rest, we often don't experience the deep restoration we seek.

Habits shape our days. Practices shape our hearts.

Both cultural and biblical rest invite us to pause, step back from work, and break the routine. But here's the difference: cultural rest disconnects to escape; biblical rest disconnects to reconnect. It's not just a break—it's a remembering of who we are and, more importantly, who God is. Historically, observing the Sabbath required deliberate planning to ensure a day set apart for rest and worship.

48 Shona Murray and David Murray, *Refresh: Embracing a Grace-Paced Life in a World of Endless Demands* (Wheaton, IL: Crossway, 2017), 54.

Many of us approach weekends with lingering to-do lists, our minds already gearing up for the coming week. This mental clutter hinders genuine rest. What if we prepared for rest as diligently as we prepared for our workweeks? What if we also prepared our meals, our homes, and our intentions for rest?

If you're anything like me, that probably sounds like more work. *I don't have a whole extra day both to prepare and to rest.* And you'd be right—we don't have the time. There's no extra day hiding in the week. But maybe that's exactly the point. There's a reason Jesus healed on the Sabbath.

Jesus didn't violate the Sabbath by healing—He revealed it. The Sabbath was never about restriction, it was always about restoration.

This kind of deep soul restoration can only come through Christ. It teaches us a heart of rest that we can then carry into our week. Rest is, at its core, a discipline of dependence.

I started this chapter with a story about how my body broke down in a place designed for health. Treadmills, supplements, and transformation plans surrounded me. But what I needed—what my body was begging for—was rest. Not the kind that comes from a nap or a vacation, but the kind that comes from surrender. I was doing all the "right" things for my health, yet I was living completely disconnected from the One who sustains it.

There is a truth that is a thread that runs through every aspect of what makes us human: dependence is foundational to health. And here we are again, full circle. Our mental, physical, and spiritual lives cannot be whole or holy without it. The Sabbath is not a spiritual luxury. It is a bodily necessity. It teaches us to let go of control and remember what's always been true: God is God, and we are not.

The world tells us to push harder, try more, optimize, and perform. But Jesus invites us to come, to lay down the burdens we were never meant to carry, and to live from a place of rest. Not passive rest, but purposeful restoration—a weekly reminder that *it is finished*, our limits are good, and our God is faithful.

In practicing rest, we aren't stepping back from health. We're stepping into it. We rehearse eternity, reorient our hearts, and renew our strength.

To do that, we must know what eternity holds—not just for our souls but our bodies. The answer will reshape how we see ourselves in light of eternity. It shifts our eyes from our own reflection to the beauty of the resurrection.

The Heart of It

Christ Connection: True rest begins with belief. The finished work of Christ reorders our hearts and reshapes our rhythms. We work from rest, not for rest.

Community Connection: When we live within our limits and practice rest, we free others to do the same and shape a culture rooted in healthy and holy rhythms.

Whole Body Connection: Rest isn't just a break, it's a practice of reconnection. By honoring the rhythms we were designed for, we embody trust and prepare our bodies and hearts for eternity.

Part 3
The Eternal Body

Real bodily hope is found only in Christ.

— Sam Allberry, *What God Has to Say about Our Bodies*

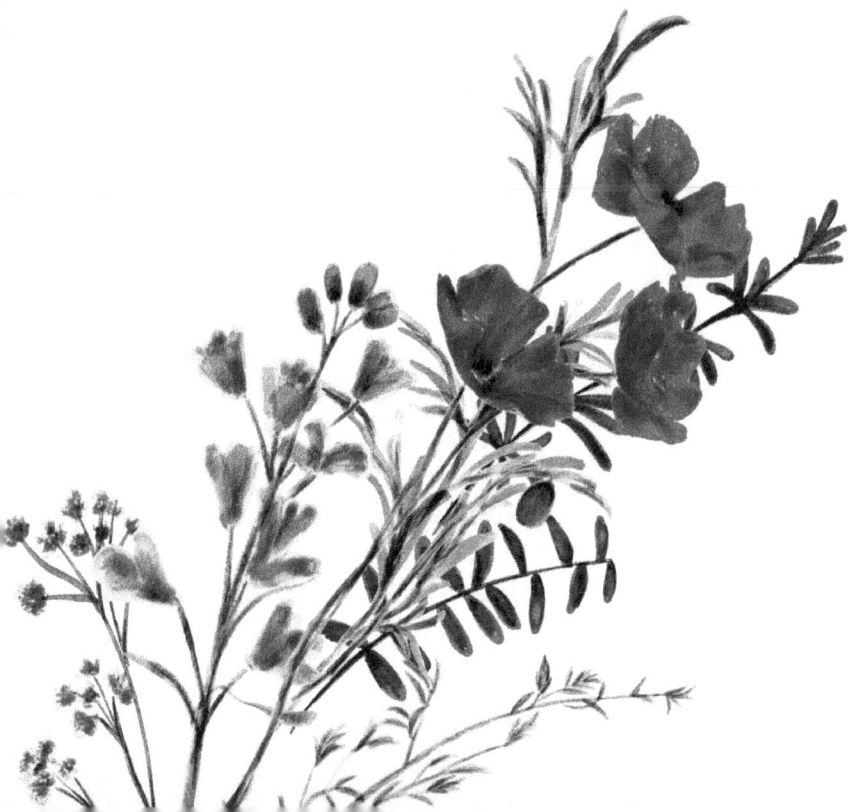

10

The Eternal Body

How does hope transform how we live in and care for our bodies?

God is not going to scrap the idea of a material world in
time and space as though He made a mistake the first time.
The biblical teaching is that God is going to restore, renew,
and re-create it, leading to a 'new heaven and a new earth'
(Isaiah 65:17; 66:22; Revelation 21:1). And God's people
will live on the new earth in resurrected bodies.

—Nancy Pearcey, *Love Thy Body*

For most of my life, I believed I was destined to struggle with my
weight. I believed it was part of my DNA.

It came from conversations I overheard—women talking
about their bodies, the rules unspoken but deeply understood. I
took notes, even as a child. Over time, this belief became a barely
conscious thought, but it shaped how I lived in my body for years.
It shaped how I moved, how I ate, how I spoke to myself in the
mirror. It was both fear and resentment—helplessness and defiant
determination, tangled together.

And now, as I age, I find a similar narrative creeping in again.
Different story. Same tone. This time, it's the signs of aging—the
subtle reminders that I can't control everything. I want to feel at
peace in my body. I want to feel at home. But I've confused peace
with ease, and comfort with control. When we place our hope in the
wrong things, we lose sight of the bigger story.

Yet the Christian story offers something else entirely. There is a
reason we declare: Hope is alive!

Our hope is not like anything else. It transcends everything.

Hope is at the heart of the Christian faith, and our hope rests in the resurrection.

But somewhere along the way, we've absorbed a version of the story missing its ending. We talk about heaven as if it's the final chapter, as if eternity is a spiritual escape where souls float free and bodies are left behind. Disembodied. Untethered. But that's not the Christian story.

Scripture doesn't end with us going *up* to heaven. It ends with heaven coming *down*. "Then I saw a new heaven and a new earth" (Revelation 21:1).

The hope of our faith isn't just that Christ died for us but that He rose. It's that *He rose in a body*. A physical, tangible, touchable body. And the promise of Scripture, the very hope we anchor ourselves to, is that what happened to Him will happen to us. Death defeated.

Bodily resurrection is not a fringe belief. It's not denominational. Across Church traditions, this is central to our faith: *we believe in the resurrection of the body*. It's not a departure from creation but a renewal of it. It's not the shedding of our bodies but their glorification. It's not an erasure but a restoration.

But why does this matter right now? We know Jesus died for our sins, and we believe in eternal life for our souls. Why does it matter that this eternal life includes a body?

Because hope isn't just about ideas. Hope becomes part of how our brains work. Over time, hope sinks into the subconscious and quietly shapes how you live in your body *now*.

Hope is the expectation of what's to come; belief is the conviction that it's already true. Hope draws us forward toward the promise of resurrection. Belief teaches us to live like it changes everything—right now. We need both. Because belief without hope feels hollow, and hope without belief drifts into wishful thinking.

Recent neuroscience confirms what the Gospel has always shown us: **hope changes the brain**. It engages the centers for motivation, goal-setting, and even healing. It builds resilience. It rewires us toward possibility.[49]

In other words, what we believe about our future shapes how we live today—even in our bodies.

Jesus's Body

When we began this journey, I suggested that the fact that Jesus rose and remains in a body is wildly significant. Why? Because this is what forms the foundation for our story. Christ's death and resurrection save us from death *through* resurrection. It's not just that He saves us; it is precisely *how* He saves us! Or, as N.T. Wright explains, "The risen Jesus is both the model for the Christian's future body and the means by which it comes about."[50]

Although there is a lot left to wonder and imagine about what it means to be in a renewed body on a new heaven and a new earth, there are some things that we can confidently build our hope in by fixing our eyes squarely upon Jesus.

First, the resurrection body was **real**. Not a spirit. Not a vision. Jesus says it plainly: "Touch me and see; a ghost does not have flesh and bones, as you see I have" (Luke 24:39). He even ate a piece of fish in front of them as if to make the point undeniable. Resurrected bodies still eat.

Jesus also **spoke** (John 20:19–21), **walked** (Luke 24:15), and **was touched** (Luke 24:39). His followers heard His voice, walked beside Him, and felt His body. The body was physical and interactive.

And then, in full view of His disciples, **He ascended** (Acts 1:9). Not shedding His body but carrying it with Him. This tells us something vital: His physicality wasn't a temporary concession. It was and is eternal.

---

49 Chan, Kee-Hyung, and Sung-Hee Shin. "The Neuroscience of Hope: Hopefulness Enhances Neuroplasticity and Stress Resilience." *Brain and Behavior* 8, no. 9 (2018): e01050. https://doi.org/10.1002/brb3.1050.

50 N.T. Wright, *Surprised by Hope: Rethinking Heaven, the Resurrection, and the Mission of the Church* (New York: HarperOne, 2008), 149.

The Apostle Paul calls Jesus the "firstfruits" of the resurrection (1 Corinthians 15:20), meaning that what happened to Him will happen to us. His resurrection is the pattern. Ours will follow.

> But as it is, Christ has been raised from the dead, the firstfruits of those who have fallen asleep.
>
> —1 Corinthians 15:20

So what does this mean for us? What kind of bodies will we have?

For years, I assumed "spiritual body" meant *only* spiritual—meaning there was nothing physical. But that's not what Paul is saying. Paul says it like this in 1 Corinthians 15:44: "Sown a natural body, raised a spiritual body. If there is a natural body, there is also a spiritual body."

Paul is teaching here that our power source, our life, will be raised to be fully united and powered by the Spirit. This doesn't mean our future bodies will be any less real. In fact, the opposite is true. As R. C. Sproul explains it, "The spiritual body is not a nonphysical body, but a body transformed by the Spirit, raised in glory, and imperishable."[51] And Wayne Grudem echoes the same idea, "Here 'spiritual' does not mean 'nonphysical,' but rather 'supernatural' and 'dominated by the Spirit.'"[52]

The future hope of eternal life is not an abstract idea. It is a real promise anchored in the real resurrection of Jesus. Hope is alive, and hope has a body!

Body of Believers

The story God is writing isn't just about individuals being restored. It's about a people made whole—a body of believers, a family.

---

51 R.C. Sproul, "Unraveling the Mystery," *Ligonier Ministries*, July 28, 2009, https://learn.ligonier.org/devotionals/unraveling-mystery.

52 Wayne Grudem, *Systematic Theology: An Introduction to Biblical Doctrine* (Grand Rapids, MI: Zondervan, 1994), 609.

If we believe that God's plan is not to scrap His creation but to redeem it, we must look at how He designed it from the start. To understand the end, we go back to the beginning. In Genesis, everything God made was good—light, land, sea, stars. But then, something wasn't. "It is not good for man to be alone."

From the beginning, relationship was central to what God declared good.

If that's how the story began, it's no surprise that our future hope isn't solitary either because our God is not solitary. He exists in perfect relationship: Father, Son, and Spirit.

Connection is not an accessory to the Christian life. It's the shape of it.

Will our relationships look different in eternity? Without a doubt. That said, we can look at some things to give us insight. In response to a Roman centurion's bold faith, Jesus says that many will come from east and west to recline at the table with Abraham, Isaac, and Jacob in the kingdom of heaven (Matthew 8:11). As Wayne Grudem points out, Jesus's mention of these patriarchs by name suggests not only that we will be *together* in eternity, but that we will be *recognizable*.[53]

Randy Alcorn makes a similar case. He points to the post-resurrection appearances of Christ, where Jesus was recognized by His disciples—not always immediately, but unmistakably.[54] The continuity was there. His body was glorified, but it was still Him. And if Christ is the firstfruits of the resurrection (1 Corinthians 15:20), then His resurrected relationships offer us a pattern, too.

Maybe you've heard this verse before and wondered what it means: "For I will create a new heavens and a new earth; the past events will not be remembered or come to mind" (Isaiah 65:17). That can feel either comforting or a little disorienting. We want to remember—especially the people we love. Part of what moves us to share the Gospel is that we want to be together for eternity, right? Most commentaries suggest that this verse doesn't mean that our

---

53 Wayne Grudem, *Systematic Theology: An Introduction to Biblical Doctrine* (Grand Rapids, MI: Zondervan, 1994), 835.

54 Randy Alcorn, *Heaven* (Carol Stream, IL: Tyndale House, 2004), 345–347.

memories will be wiped clean, but that our memories, instead, will be cleansed and restored.[55]

How great is that? Community, togetherness, a people, and a *body* for eternity. And of course, we should not be surprised to find that the Gospel story is never one of separation. It's a story of connection.

Eternal Body

We long to be with the people we love, but we also long to still be ourselves. That's often the unspoken question beneath our hope for eternity: *Will I still be me?*

That same verse in Isaiah may also lead some of us to believe we won't remember who we are. Will we just be absorbed into eternity, where we cease to exist? I am sometimes scared to ask these questions because I don't want it to appear as if I am suggesting that God isn't enough. But I also don't long for an eternity where I cease to be, well … me. Free from pain, yes, but also free from form and identity.

This is why what we believe about eternity matters here and now. If we don't believe that eternity holds something good, we'll be tempted to place our hope in lesser things. Things that distract us from the One who offers true hope. So, who are we in light of eternity? Once again, we fix our eyes on Jesus to discover what is true.

The idea of continuity is affirmed by many biblical scholars across traditions. Jesus did not receive a different body. He received His own body, made new. This matters. Because it means that our future selves will still be ourselves. Not erased, not replaced, but redeemed. This is why what we do now in these bodies matters for eternity.

In *Systematic Theology*, Wayne Grudem presents a clear case for continuity between our current bodies and our resurrection bodies. He explains that Paul uses the image of a seed in the ground to

55 "Will We Remember Our Lives in Heaven?" *Got Questions Ministries*, accessed April 14, 2025, https://www.gotquestions.org/remember-Heaven.html.

> What you sow does not come to life unless it dies. And as for what you sow—you are not sowing a body that will be, but only a seed, perhaps of wheat or another grain. But God gives it a body as he wants, and to each of the seeds its own body.
>
> —1 Corinthians 15:36-38

describe the resurrection (1 Corinthians 15:36–38). A seed doesn't disappear. It changes. What grows is connected to what was planted. They are different in form but the same in essence.

Jesus's body bore the marks of His suffering. The scars were not erased. He invited Thomas to see and touch them (John 20:27). His resurrected body wasn't replaced; it was renewed. Transformed, yes—but still His. That's no small detail. And yet, it was also unlike anything anyone had seen before. He appeared in locked rooms. At times, He was not immediately recognized—Mary mistook Him for the gardener (John 20:15), and the disciples on the road to Emmaus didn't realize who He was until He broke bread (Luke 24:16, 30–31). But eventually, they all saw Him clearly. His body was changed and glorified, but it was still His.[56]

Although I can't say which scars we'll carry into eternity, it comforts me that the hard-fought, wrestled-through parts of our story—the ones that shape who we are—don't just fall away. When we use our bodies for kingdom purposes, it seems they go with us. Not erased, but carried forward. Transformed. Fulfilled.

N.T. Wright says it like this: "All we can surmise from the picture of Jesus's resurrection is that just as his wounds were still visible, not now as a source of pain and death but as signs of victory, so the Christian's risen body will bear such marks of his or her loyalty to

---

56 Wayne Grudem, *Systematic Theology: An Introduction to Biblical Doctrine* (Grand Rapids, MI: Zondervan, 1994), 831–836.

God's particular calling as are appropriate, not the least where that has involved suffering."[57]

Our bodies are not forgotten. They are sown in faith-like seeds and raised in glory, like Christ.

We live in these bodies with the end in view.

Our hope is in something so miraculous, so extraordinary, that it can feel distant from daily life. But the people we are now, in these bodies, are the ones Christ redeems. The work we do to care for them, the choices we make, the grace we receive, and the way we keep showing up are not wasted. It carries into eternity. There is continuity. Glory doesn't start after. It begins now. The resurrection gives us vision—to see our whole selves with eternal eyes.

The Heart of It

Christ Connection: The resurrection of Jesus is both the means of our salvation and the mirror of our future. His glorified body tells the whole story—our story.

Community Connection: Resurrection is reunion. We are not saved into solitude but into a body, where recognition, relationship, and restoration continue forever.

Whole Body Connection: What we do in these bodies matters. They are not temporary containers but eternal seeds—sown in faith, raised in glory, and formed for forever.

---

57 N. T. Wright, *Surprised by Hope: Rethinking Heaven, the Resurrection, and the Mission of the Church* (New York: HarperOne, 2008), 160.

11

Body Image

How does the Gospel transform how we see our bodies?

Through our bodies we relate to others. Through our bodies we learn who we are. Through our bodies we live fully in the world God created.

—Paula Gooder, *Body*

The Gospel really is the answer to everything. Had you told me 10 years ago that it could change the way I saw my body, I would have agreed with you, but I wouldn't have believed you. It would have sounded nice, but I would have searched for the answers in the next bit of research. I would have continued to obsess over what I saw in the mirror, comparing my body, my hair, my skin, to everyone else selling a product with the promise of health, beauty, youth, and fitness.

But I am now sold on something else. I am sold on the reality that when we truly fix our eyes on Christ, seek first the kingdom of God, and choose to walk in His ways and not our own, we will find a new set of answers—*better* answers. A solution that doesn't require us to waste our money and time on products chasing a temporary view of beauty and health. When we stop looking for answers in the mirror, we're finally free to see what's true. Not just about our bodies, but about the One who made them.

We begin to see our bodies for what they are: holy ground.

And we begin to see a new kind of mirror. One that is a place of truth, not torment. Kyle Worley calls Christ the "true mirror", and describes it like this, "It is the best kind of honest assessment, the kind that shows us our imperfections while never once calling into question who God has declared us to be."[58]

In other words, when we look to Jesus, we can see ourselves the way God sees us. And over time, we stop trying to look like the world and start looking more like Him.

Here is the remarkable truth. **You are united with Christ.**

His body was broken, so yours could truly live. He is with you, and you are with Him. You don't have to fight for worth. Or prove your value. Or fix yourself. You are already home.

Union with Christ doesn't mean you'll never wrestle with body image again. It means you'll never wrestle alone.

You are at home in your body because you are at home in Him.

Because to be united with Christ is to be united with Him and His body—made whole in Him. Our union with Christ is the thread that ties it all together.

I hope we continue the conversation about how God designed our bodies to thrive with care, wisdom, and intention. But I've learned that we often rush to the *how-to* of health before considering what we need and *Who* we need. Before the habits, we sometimes need a heart-to-heart. Before we act, we need to remember who we are.

Health is an outworking of His grace and goodness through our efforts. And while this book has centered on the heart and mind, I hope we keep going. I hope we talk more about rhythms of nourishment, rest, movement, and the kind of care that aligns with God's creation, not just cultural trends, because caring for the body matters deeply.

But all that flows from this starting point: a desire to honor what God has declared good. A desire to embody what we believe. A desire to connect with God, His people, and His creation through our bodies.

---

58 Kyle Worley, *Home with God: A Guide to Knowing and Enjoying Him* (Nashville: B&H Publishing, 2023), 124.

I have reflected a lot on the man in John chapter 5 who had been disabled for thirty-eight years, waiting by the pool of Bethesda, hoping for a chance to step into waters he believed would heal him. I have read a ton of commentaries on this section of Scripture, and there are varying takes on why Jesus would ask him a question to which the answer seems so obvious, "Do you want to get well?".

His nearness to the pool seems to say it all. Of course, he wants to get well. Why else would he be there waiting by the waters he believed would bring restoration? However, it wasn't until that desire was brought to Jesus that everything changed. I wonder if, in that moment, the man realized he had been drawing near to the wrong source of life all along.

I sometimes take for granted that God knows my struggles, and I forget that connection happens through my communication to Him. Prayer reminds me of who I am and who He is. God sent His Son in a body, to live in a body, to suffer in a body, to die in a body, and to be resurrected in a body so that we could follow Him.

Where do we go from here? I love the quote from Lara Casey: "Prayer is an action step, friend."[59] We start where we are. We pray. Gratitude, dependence, and presence are wrapped into one simple, humble act. It never feels like enough, but it is our greatest superpower.

No book or system can tell you what God is calling you to. I don't know what gifts he has given to you or what your family needs. I don't know what has happened to your body. I don't know what obstacles you have had to overcome, and I don't know in what ways you may need to go out of your way to give your body something it needs right now. The world is noisy. I know it can feel incredibly overwhelming, especially to women. I have been in the health and fitness world long enough to see the trends come and go. But this is why we must root ourselves firmly in the One who doesn't change.

So we begin there. With prayer. Not as a last resort but as our first act of connection.

59 Lara Casey, *Make It Happen: Surrender Your Fear. Take the Leap. Live on Purpose.* (Nashville: Thomas Nelson, 2014), 48.

100

It's not connection to a method or a system, but to the God who made us—who knit us together, body and soul, and called it good.

We don't start by fixing ourselves. We start by turning toward Him.

Sometimes the most faithful thing we can do is stop long enough to ask honest questions in the presence of God. Not to find the perfect answer but to return and remember.

What cultural standards am I still holding onto? How are they shaping my relationship with my body?

What does my body need in this season—rest, nourishment, movement?

Where might God be inviting me to simplify so I can be more present?

Where am I sensing disconnection from God, from others, or even from myself? What might it look like to move toward reconnection?

I grew up in the era of WWJD bracelets. Who doesn't love a fashion trend that doubles as spiritual formation? A little cheesy, maybe—but also clarifying. What would Jesus do? We know what He did. We have His words. We've seen how He lived, how He moved, how He related to the Father.

In Jesus's body, we find the storyline of our own.

So we follow Him, not just in belief but in embodiment. We care for our bodies not to chase perfection but to live in a deeper connection to God, others, and ourselves. To be whole means to no longer live fragmented—torn between what we believe and how we live, between what we know is true and what we feel in our bodies. It means heart, mind, soul, and will moving together, aligned in truth. **Wholeness is not perfection. It is integrity. It is when our beliefs are not just something we think but something we carry out through our bodies.**

To be holy means to be set apart, not by making ourselves good, but by belonging fully to the One who is. It's about not conforming to the cultural climate but instead being shaped by an eternal kingdom.

Holiness does not isolate us from the world. It anchors us in God's presence as we move through it. It is the confidence of a life that is not self-made, but Spirit-formed.

> **Therefore, whether we are at home or away, we make it our aim to be pleasing to him.**
> **—2 Corinthians 5:9**

A Gospel-shaped body is both whole and holy. It is to live connected and set apart—body and soul, earth and heaven, now and forever.

Paul says that "while we are at home in the body, we are away from the Lord" (2 Corinthians 5:6), not because the body isn't good, but because we await something better. We live in that tension.

The more we live by faith, anchored in eternal things, the more at home we are. Not because our bodies have changed, but we are learning to live embodied, and in light of eternity through the full message of the Gospel.

It's not about doing more. It's about living from what has already been done. I can tell you how Jesus changes everything, but to encounter it, you have to embody it. It's worship. It's relationship. It's living with your whole heart, mind, and body. It's the most beautiful life you could ever hope for.

Through Christ, we always find our way back home.

Thank You

To my mom for sharing the Gospel with me—the greatest gift I've ever received.

To my husband for your support. Thank you for reading every word, and for loving me enough to tell the truth, even when it meant starting over.

To Alex Ford, your wisdom and friendship have shaped this message more than you know. I read everything you recommend, and I'm grateful your insight found its way into these pages.

To Alli Worthington for your encouragement and wisdom that always keeps me moving forward. Your mentorship is a gift.

Sources

Part 1

Kapic, Kelly M. *You're Only Human: How Your Limits Reflect God's Design and Why That's Good News.* Grand Rapids, MI: Brazos Press, 2022.

Chapter 1 Sources:

Allberry, Sam. *What God Has to Say About Our Bodies: How the Gospel Is Good News for Our Physical Selves.* Wheaton, IL: Crossway, 2021

1. Runfola, Cristin D., Ann Von Holle, Kimberly A. Peat, Nancy Zucker, and Cynthia M. Bulik. "Characteristics of Women with Body Size Satisfaction at Midlife: Results of the Gender and Body Image (GABI) Study." *Journal of Women & Aging* 25, no. 4 (2013): 287–304. https://doi.org/10.1080/08952841.2013.816215.

2. Wood, Joanne V., W. Q. Elaine Perunovic, and John W. Lee. "Positive Self-Statements: Power for Some, Peril for Others." *Psychological Science* 20, no. 7 (2009): 860–866. https://doi.org/10.1111/j.1467-9280.2009.02370.x.

Chapter 2 Sources:

Pearcey, Nancy R. *Love Thy Body: Answering Hard Questions about Life and Sexuality.* Grand Rapids, MI: Baker Books, 2018.

3. Solfrid Bratland-Sanda, Merethe Pauline Nilsson, and Jorunn Sundgot-Borgen, "Disordered Eating Behavior Among Group Fitness Instructors: A Health-Threatening Secret?" *Journal of Eating Disorders* 3, no. 22 (2015), https://doi.org/10.1186/s40337-015-0059-x.

4. Crain, Natasha. "Practical Tips for Teaching Kids Apologetics at Home." *The Natasha Crain Podcast.* August 24, 2021. Audio, 1:16:00. https://podcasts.apple.com/us/podcast/practical-tips-for-teaching-kids-apologetics-at-home/id1550242146?i=1000532918332.

5. Crain, Natasha. *Faithfully Different: Regaining Biblical Clarity in a Secular Culture.* Harvest House Publishers, 2022

6. Barna Group. "Most Adults Feel Accepted by God, but Lack a Biblical Worldview." *Barna.* March 6, 2005. https://www.barna.com/research/most-adults-feel-accepted-by-god-but-lack-a-biblical-worldview/.

7. Wiersbe, Warren W. *The Bible Exposition Commentary.* Wheaton, IL: Victor Books, 1989.

8. Kite, Lexie, and Lindsay Kite. *More Than a Body: Your Body Is an Instrument, Not an Ornament.* Boston: Houghton Mifflin Harcourt, 2021.

9. Pearcey, Nancy R. *Love Thy Body: Answering Hard Questions about Life and Sexuality.* Grand Rapids, MI: Baker Books, 2018.

10. Simons, Ruth Chou. *Pilgrim: 25 Ways God's Character Leads Us Onward.* Nashville: Harvest House Publishers, 2023.

11. Blue Letter Bible. "H2896 - tôb - Strong's Hebrew Lexicon." Accessed May 9, 2025. https://www.blueletterbible.org/lexicon/h2896/kjv/wlc/0-1/.

12. Stott, John R. W. *The Message of the Sermon on the Mount.* Downers Grove, IL: InterVarsity Press, 1978.

Chapter 3 Sources:

Caldecott, Stratford. *Beauty for Truth's Sake: On the Re-enchantment of Education.* Grand Rapids, MI: Brazos Press, 2009.

13. MarketResearch.com. "U.S. Weight Loss Industry Grows to $90 Billion, Fueled by Obesity Drugs Demand." *MarketResearch.com.* April 10, 2023. https://blog.marketresearch.com/u.s.-weight-loss-industry-grows-to-90-billion-fueled-by-obesity-drugs-demand.

14. McKinsey & Company. "The Beauty Market in 2023: A Special State of Fashion Report." *McKinsey & Company.* May 4, 2023. https://www.mckinsey.com/industries/retail/our-insights/the-beauty-market-in-2023-a-special-state-of-fashion-report.

15. Crain, Natasha. *Talking with Your Kids about Jesus: 30 Conversations Every Christian Parent Must Have*. Minneapolis: Bethany House, 2020.

Chapter 4 Sources:

Warren, Tish Harrison. *Liturgy of the Ordinary: Sacred Practices in Everyday Life*. Downers Grove, IL: InterVarsity Press, 2016.

16. *Blue Letter Bible*. "Matthew 4 – Greek Lexicon." https://www.blueletterbible.org/csb/mat/4/1/t_conc_933001.

  Blue Letter Bible. "Mark 1 – Greek Lexicon." https://www.blueletterbible.org/csb/mar/1/12/t_conc_958012.

  Blue Letter Bible. "Luke 4 – Greek Lexicon." https://www.blueletterbible.org/csb/luk/4/1/t_conc_977001

17. Paula Gooder, *Body: Biblical Spirituality for the Whole Person* (London: SPCK, 2016), 109.

18. Kapic, Kelly M. *You're Only Human: How Your Limits Reflect God's Design and Why That's Good News*. Grand Rapids, MI: Brazos Press, 2022.

19. Mineo, Liz. "Over Nearly 80 Years, Harvard Study Has Been Showing How to Live a Healthy and Happy Life." *Harvard Gazette*. April 11, 2017. https://news.harvard.edu/gazette/story/2017/04/over-nearly-80-years-harvard-study-has-been-showing-how-to-live-a-healthy-and-happy-life/.

20. Heitzig, Skip. *Bloodline: Tracing God's Rescue Plan from Eden to Eternity*. Colorado Springs: Worthy Publishing, 2018.

21. Lewis, C. S. *The Problem of Pain*. New York: HarperOne, 2001.

Chapter 5 Sources:

Wirzba, Norman. *Food and Faith: A Theology of Eating*. New York: Cambridge University Press, 2011.

22. Harris, Emily. "Meta-Analysis: Social Isolation, Loneliness Tied to Higher Mortality." *JAMA* 330, no. 3 (July 18, 2023): 211. https://jamanetwork.com/journals/jama/article-abstract/2806852.

23. Finley, Anna J., and Stacey M. Schaefer. "Affective Neuroscience of Loneliness: Potential Mechanisms Underlying the Association Between Perceived Social Isolation, Health, and Well-Being." *Journal of Psychiatric and Brain Science* 7, no. 6 (December 26, 2022): e220011. https://doi.org/10.20900/jpbs.20220011.

24. Yu, Xuexin, Tsai-Chin Cho, Ashly C. Westrick, Chen Chen, Kenneth M. Langa, and Lindsay C. Kobayashi. "Association of Cumulative Loneliness with All-Cause Mortality among Middle-Aged and Older Adults in the United States, 1996 to 2019." *Proceedings of the National Academy of Sciences* 120, no. 51 (December 11, 2023): e2306819120. https://doi.org/10.1073/pnas.2306819120.

25. Reinke, Tony. *12 Ways Your Phone Is Changing You*. Wheaton, IL: Crossway, 2017.

26. Crain, Natasha. *Faithfully Different: Regaining Biblical Clarity in a Secular Culture*. Minneapolis: Bethany House, 2022.

Part 2

Warren, Tish Harrison. *Liturgy of the Ordinary: Sacred Practices in Everyday Life*. Downers Grove, IL: InterVarsity Press, 2016.

Chapter 6 Sources:

Stone, Rachel Marie. *Eat with Joy: Redeeming God's Gift of Food*. Downers Grove, IL: InterVarsity Press, 2013.

27. Froreich, Franzisca V., Lenny R. Vartanian, Matthew J. Zawadzki, Jessica R. Grisham, and Stephen W. Touyz. "Psychological Need Satisfaction, Control, and Disordered Eating." *British Journal of Clinical Psychology* 56, no. 1 (March 2017): 53–68. https://doi.org/10.1111/bjc.12120.

28. Morin, Amy. "7 Scientifically Proven Benefits of Gratitude." *Psychology Today*, April 3, 2015. https://www.psychologytoday.com/us/blog/what-mentally-strong-people-dont-do/201504/7-scientifically-proven-benefits-of-gratitude.

29. Jacob, H.E. *Six Thousand Years of Bread: Its Holy and Unholy History.* New York: Lyons Press, 1944.

Wirzba, Norman. *Food and Faith: A Theology of Eating.* New York: Cambridge University Press, 2011.

30. Earley, Justin Whitmel. *The Common Rule: Habits of Purpose for an Age of Distraction.* Downers Grove, IL: InterVarsity Press, 2019

31. Haines, Jess, Katherine W. Norris, Maha Obeid, Yvonne Fu, Michael Weinstangel, and Thomas Sampson. "Systematic Review of the Effects of Family Meal Frequency on Psychosocial Outcomes in Youth." *Canadian Family Physician* 61, no. 2 (February 2015): e96–e106. https://www.ncbi.nlm.nih.gov/pmc/articles/PMC4325878/.

32. Rachel Marie Stone, *Eat with Joy: Redeeming God's Gift of Food* (Downers Grove, IL: InterVarsity Press, 2013), 67.

33. Erickson, Jamie. *Holy Hygge: Creating a Place for People to Gather and the Gospel to Grow.* Chicago: Moody Publishers, 2022.

Chapter 7 Sources:

Carlson, Lindsey. *Identity Theft: Reclaiming the Truth of Our Identity in Christ.* Wheaton, IL: Crossway, 2019.

34. Fahmy, Sam. "Low-Intensity Exercise Reduces Fatigue Symptoms by 65 Percent, Study Finds." *UGA Today*, February 28, 2008. https://news.uga.edu/low-intensity-exercise-reduces-fatigue-symptoms-by-65-percent-study-finds/.

35. Statista. "Energy Drinks – Worldwide." *Statista Research Department.* Accessed March 29, 2025. https://www.statista.com/topics/10313/energy-drinks-worldwide/.

36. Allied Market Research. *Energy Supplement Market.* August 2022. https://www.alliedmarketresearch.com/energy-supplement-market-A16879.

37. Brown, Nick. "Report: Daily U.S. Coffee Consumption Hits 20-Year High." *Daily Coffee News.* April 12, 2024. https://dailycoffee-news.com/2024/04/12/report-daily-us-coffee-consumption-hits-20-year-high/.

38. Yorks, Dayna M., Christopher A. Frothingham, and Mark D. Schuenke. "Effects of Group Fitness Classes on Stress and Quality of Life of Medical Students." *Journal of the American Osteopathic Association* 117, no. 11 (November 2017): e17–e25. https://doi.org/10.7556/jaoa.2017.140.

39. Estabrooks, P.A. "Sustaining Exercise Participation Through Group Cohesion." *Exercise and Sport Sciences Reviews* 28, no. 2 (April 2000): 63–67. https://pubmed.ncbi.nlm.nih.gov/10902087/.

40. Means, Casey, MD, and Calley Means. *Good Energy: The Surprising Connection Between Metabolism and Limitless Health.* New York: Avery Publishing Group, 2024.

Chapter 8 Sources:

Lyons, Rebekah. *Building a Resilient Life: How Adversity Awakens Strength, Hope, and Meaning.* Grand Rapids, MI: Zondervan, 2023.

41. *Bible Hub.* HELPS Word-Studies. S.v. "Merimnaó (Strong's 3309)." https://biblehub.com/greek/3309.htm.

42. Coutu, Diane L. "How Resilience Works." *Harvard Business Review* 80, no. 5 (May 2002): 46–50, 52, 55. https://hbr.org/2002/05/how-resilience-works.

43. Schnall, Simone, Kent D. Harber, Jeanine K. Stefanucci, and Dennis R. Proffitt. "Social Support and the Perception of Geographical Slant." *Journal of Experimental Social Psychology* 43, no. 5 (September 2008): 1246–1255. https://doi.org/10.1016/j.jesp.2008.04.011.

44. Ko, Stephen. *Faith Embodied.* Grand Rapids, MI: Zondervan, 2025.

45. Simons, Ruth Chou. *Now and Not Yet: Pressing in When You're Waiting, Wanting, and Restless for More.* Nashville: Thomas Nelson, 2024.

Chapter 9 Sources:

Buchanan, Mark. *The Rest of God: Restoring Your Soul by Restoring Sabbath.* Nashville: Thomas Nelson, 2006.

46. Shanafelt, Tait, et al. "Changes in Burnout and Satisfaction With Work-Life Integration in Physicians and the General US Working Population Between 2011 and 2021." *JAMA Network Open 5*, no. 11 (November 2022): e2239346. https://doi.org/10.1001/jamanetworkopen.2022.39346.

47. Kuroda, Sachiko, and Isamu Yamamoto. "Does Overwork Decrease Productivity? Evidence from Panel Data on Japanese Workers." *Scandinavian Journal of Work, Environment & Health* 49, no. 2 (2023): 138–146. https://doi.org/10.5271/sjweh.4066.

48. Murray, Shona, and David Murray. *Refresh: Embracing a Grace-Paced Life in a World of Endless Demands.* Wheaton, IL: Crossway, 2017.

Part 3

Allberry, Sam. *What God Has to Say About Our Bodies: How the Gospel Is Good News for Our Physical Selves.* Wheaton, IL: Crossway, 2021.

Chapter 10 Sources:

Pearcey, Nancy. *Love Thy Body: Answering Hard Questions About Life and Sexuality.* Grand Rapids, MI: Baker Books, 2018.

49. Chan, Kee-Hyung, and Sung-Hee Shin. "The Neuroscience of Hope: Hopefulness Enhances Neuroplasticity and Stress Resilience." *Brain and Behavior* 8, no. 9 (2018): e01050. https://doi.org/10.1002/brb3.1050.

50. Wright, N.T. *Surprised by Hope: Rethinking Heaven, the Resurrection, and the Mission of the Church.* New York: HarperOne, 2008.

51. Sproul, R.C. Unraveling the Mystery. *Ligonier Ministries,* July 28, 2009. https://learn.ligonier.org/devotionals/unraveling-mystery.

52. Grudem, Wayne. *Systematic Theology: An Introduction to Biblical Doctrine.* Grand Rapids, MI: Zondervan, 1994. Wikipedia+2theoutlet. us+2Truth Story+2

53. Grudem, Wayne. *Systematic Theology: An Introduction to Biblical Doctrine.* Grand Rapids, MI: Zondervan, 1994.

54. Alcorn, Randy. *Heaven.* Carol Stream, IL: Tyndale House, 2004.

55. Got Questions Ministries. "Will We Remember Our Lives in Heaven?" Accessed April 14, 2025. https://www.gotquestions.org/remember-Heaven.html.

56. Grudem, Wayne. *Systematic Theology: An Introduction to Biblical Doctrine.* Grand Rapids, MI: Zondervan, 1994.

57. Wright, N. T. *Surprised by Hope: Rethinking Heaven, the Resurrection, and the Mission of the Church.* New York: HarperOne, 2008.

Chapter 11 Sources:

Gooder, Paula. *Body: Biblical Spirituality for the Whole Person.* Grand Rapids: Baker Academic, 2016.

58. Worley, Kyle. *Home with God: A Guide to Knowing and Enjoying Him.* Nashville: B&H Publishing, 2023.

59. Casey, Lara. *Make It Happen: Surrender Your Fear. Take the Leap. Live on Purpose.* Nashville: Thomas Nelson, 2014.

www.ingramcontent.com/pod-product-compliance
Lightning Source LLC
Chambersburg PA
CBHW031542260326
41914CB00002B/227